Copyright © 2021 Nicole Eichinger

All rights reserved. No part of this publication may be reproduced without the prior written consent of the copyright holder, except in the case of brief quotations for reviewing purposes.

Cover and Interior Design: Nicole Eichinger
Editor: Anna Nelson anna@osswriting.com
Back Cover Photo: David Eichinger
Interior Layout: Homestead Publishing Co. www.homesteadpublishingco.com

Nicole Eichinger is a Registered Dietitian.

Nicole received her Bachelor of Science in
Nutritional Science from
Texas Tech University,
did her dietetic Internship with ARAMARK Kansas City,
worked as a Neonatal Intensive Care & Pediatric Dietitian,
worked as a home therapy Renal Dietitian and
then started her own business: Nutrition's My Life.

The Healthy Thyroid Guide is not to be copied or distributed.
The Healthy Thyroid Guide is not to be taken as medical
advice but as a resource for educational purposes.

Dedicated to:

My husband who supports my dreams and loves me entirely.
My kids who look up to me and keep me on my toes.
My parents and siblings who have believed in me my entire life.
My editor who helped make this book surpass my dreams.
And
All the thyroid warriors who have struggled for too long.

Healthy Thyroid Guide

The thyroid influences almost every cell in the body, which means the entire body must be addressed to improve it's health. Thyroid health is complex and confusing for many. I know for many years I felt crazy. I'd go to the doctors exhausted with heart palpitations. The doctor would always say, "Your labs look great." But I still felt bad.

You've probably had similar feelings or thoughts. Things did not start to turn around for me until I understood what my body needed. I'm honored to be able to provide you with the tools in this guide to help you along your thyroid journey.

I developed this *Healthy Thyroid Guide* for ALL thyroid warriors. If you have hyperthyroid, hypothyroid, NO thyroid, thyroid cancer, thyroid nodules/tumors or autoimmune disorders such as Hashimoto's or Graves' disease, this guide is designed for you!

I knew that if I, a registered dietitian, was struggling with my thyroid health, even when I ate healthy, that the general public must be really struggling! This guide stems from my experience, but it is here to provide you with the science behind why these tools work! My tips have already helped thousands of people, and I am excited to share them with you now, too!

Healthy Thyroid Guide

Table of Contents

My Thyroid Story 8

Chapter One: What's the Thyroid's Job and How Does It Work? ... 27

Chapter Two: Different Thyroid Disorders 43

Chapter Three: Thyroid Hormones and Labs 59

Chapter Four: Lifestyle Factors 67

Chapter Five: Thyroid Challenges Part One

    – Cortisol, Estrogen, Menstrual Cycles, Menopause, Men, and Transgender 79

Chapter Six: Thyroid Challenges Part Two

    – Weight Loss, Sleep, Stress, and Hair loss 97

Chapter Seven: Thyroid Supporting Nutrients 121

Chapter Eight: Nutrition Confusion 161

Chapter Nine: How to Eat for Your Thyroid 175

Chapter Ten: Thyroid Supplements 187

Chapter Eleven: Recipes 191

Chapter Twelve: Feel Good Food Diary and Non-negotiables 217

Notes 240

References 244

Healthy Thyroid Guide

My Thyroid Story

This book is my guide to help you improve your thyroid health through diet, exercise, and lifestyle choice. But first, let me tell you what makes me uniquely qualified to be your guide. As a registered dietitian with half a thyroid, I am able to bring you my real life experiences as well as the science behind improving your health with a thyroid disorder. I understand what you're going through because I've been there myself. I'm also specially trained to understand how to make the thyroid (or thyroid medication) work at it's optimal level. I feel called to share my health history and journey with you.

Here's my story:

My thyroid story starts when I was in high school. I was an elite soccer, player living my best life, until I ran into some serious injuries. It all started when I was trying to steal the ball back from my opponent. In the heat of the game, I put my arm out to move her out of the way. Suddenly, I felt the back of my hand hit my back and a lot of pain in my arm.

I initially thought I dislocated my elbow. It was not until I got to the hospital that I found I had a spiral fracture to my right humerus (the big bone in the upper arm).

My Thyroid Story

It took four hours in the Emergency Room for the doctors to try to set my arm They had to manipulate the bones to get them to line up and, during this time, they had me in a continuous x-ray machine. I was exposed to a lot of radiation that day. Afterward, my arm was not healing well, so I received even more x-rays on and off for nine months (as you can imagine, all this caused a lot of both emotional and physical stress).

The healing journey for my arm was a slow and painful one. I had to sleep sitting up for four months because I couldn't bear the pain while lying down. My arm was struggling to heal; therefore, I had to wear a bone stimulator to bed for three months. Even after my broken humerus healed, I eventually needed shoulder surgery because my ligaments/tendons stretched while being in a sling for so long (this added more emotional and physical stress).

Four months after my arm/shoulder healed, I was back to playing soccer again and was the happiest girl! However, in my first game back one of the opponent's teammates and I went for the ball at the same time near midfield. I twisted wrong and pop, pop, pop, pop! My knee injury was so loud that, the goalkeeper heard could hear my tearing ligaments as I went down. I tore four ligaments in my left knee and needed surgery.

My Thyroid Story

After yet another nine months of healing, I was ready to get back into the game. I trained all summer, with my amazing father acting as my endurance coach. And, because of our hard work, I was healthy enough to play soccer at the university of my choice. I chose Texas Tech and was thrilled to join their team.

To play Division 1 soccer at Texas Tech, I had to get a very in-depth physical. During it, the doctor felt my neck and asked, "Have you always had this lump in your throat?" This was the beginning of my thyroid journey. The doctor obtained a biopsy of the lump and it was found to be pre-cancerous. The doctor recommended a right partial thyroidectomy or removal of the right side of the thyroid that had gotten significantly larger than the left side. I underwent surgery and will always remember my mom being there for me. We strongly believe the x-ray radiation to my right arm and the continual stress/trauma was what caused the right side of my thyroid to grow abnormal cells (and bring on yet another time of high emotional and physical stress for me).

I was seven hours away from my parents, playing soccer, studying, and slowly dipping into a depression because of my new medical issues, but I didn't know it at the time.

My Thyroid Story

As a naive 20-year-old, I did not know I needed to see an endocrinologist after losing half my thyroid. No one told me to do labs. No one told me the reason I was experiencing crazy mood swings, depression, and anxiety was because I went from having a full thyroid with full thyroid hormones to only half a thyroid. My body was experiencing a hormonal shift but I wasn't receiving help to adjust to the change. No one told me the anti-depressant and the anti-anxiety medications I was prescribed would just be a band-aid and I'd still feel exhausted all the time. My root cause to all my problems was never addressed.

It was not until two years after the right side of my thyroid was removed that I was referred to an endocrinologist who finally placed me on thyroid hormone replacement medication.

I remember the doctor telling me, "This little pill has to be taken every day but think of it as your set metabolism for life!"

I thought to myself, "I'm actually really lucky!!" I was under the impression I would not ever have to worry about my weight, and I was happy about it at first! I felt like I had an advantage over most people... wow, was I ever wrong.

My Thyroid Story

No one told me that you can still have hypothyroid symptoms while on your thyroid replacement medication. No one told me I would have a roller coaster of mood swings. No one told me I'd be completely exhausted just by a normal day of work. No one told me I would have heart palpitations or that my thyroid and menstrual cycles were related. No one told me anything but "your labs look good."

I felt like I always came up empty handed when I asked for helped at my doctors appointments. I was tired of not getting anywhere, I started searching for answers of my own but it may not be where you think.

I had an awesome job when I started my career as a dietitian. I worked in the Neonatal Intensive Care Unit (NICU) and I absolutely loved it! It was hard work: I had to think on my feet, I had to be good with math, and I had to understand the body on a very complex level. My love for digestive health started in the NICU with a little baby, we'll call her Amera.

Baby Amera was born with multiple medical issues – from cardiac problems to short bowel syndrome, to blindness and even fluid on the brain. She also had a lot of people who watched out for her. My job was to help her heal after her many surgeries, to help keep her alive, and to help her grow.

My Thyroid Story

I looked forward to visiting her every day, to see her beautiful, crooked smile

What was extremely challenging for this baby's team was her massive diarrhea blowouts. She struggled to digest her formula properly. So, I had to get to know this baby. I grew to understand her and to understand that what she was telling me through her symptoms and labs was that her specialized formula was not working. We tried multiple different specialized formulas provided by the hospital but she just did not tolerate any of them. I could not give up, though, because her life would be so much better if she could just absorb and tolerate her nutrition.

It was up to me to make a customized baby formula just for her. I used oils from the kitchen for her fat intake, we designed a hypoallergenic formula (which means there were no preservatives and all ingredients were broken down in their smallest form) and I added EXTRA nutrients to help her based on her specific needs.

She started getting better. She began tolerating her feedings and eventually became a happy baby, healthy enough that she could start playing on her own. Her quality of life improved because her body was finally receiving the nutrition it needed.

My Thyroid Story

This first real challenge sent my love for digestion into high gear, and I found I was good at figuring out its mysteries. I was really good at my job. I started getting more and more referrals from the physicians for my help. I worked in an on-call rotation with other dietitians to cover late evenings and weekend. I had just gotten married, bought a house and after three years of working in the NICU I got pregnant. It was an exciting time until I had an extremely traumatic birth with my daughter.

When I say traumatic, I mean I had a 104°F fever. My placenta was infected; therefore, the contractions were unbearable and felt like knives sticking into my abdomen and back.

I had to bear the pain because the epidurals, yes plural, weren't working. In the fourth hour of active pushing and eighteenth hours of active labor, I didn't notice as the nurses posted up on stools next to me because I was so exhausted I was falling asleep in between pushes. Turns out, they moved in close just in case they needed to break my pelvis because my daughter was stuck with her meconium inside me *(are you seeing the trend... here's even more emotional and physical stress in my life).*

My Thyroid Story

After her birth, I worked as much as I could and tried to be the best "Pinterest" mom I could be! (You know, the DIY, everything from scratch, and put way more stress on yourself than is necessary-mom.) I would workout hard, sleep only a little, but at least I had my meal prepping to keep things going for me.

Pretty soon, I realized I had to find a new job because my hours at the NICU were unrealistic for me as a parent. I would come home from work and collapse on the floor out of exhaustion. I had to make some changes.

It started with finding a new job and cutting my work down to only 24 hours a week. In the first week of working at the new company we had a mandatory dietitian meeting. Unfortunately, I miscarried the morning of the meeting. I was brand new to this position with no time off, so the only logical thing I could think to do was to just wear a pad and go into the meeting *(another emotional and physical stressful time)*.

Somehow, I survived the meeting and felt blessed when I ended up pregnant again the very next month. This time I had a healthy pregnancy and a better delivery than I did with my daughter. I went back to work after 12 weeks at home with my son and worked the full 32 hours I was allotted. But, it only lasted a few years.

My Thyroid Story

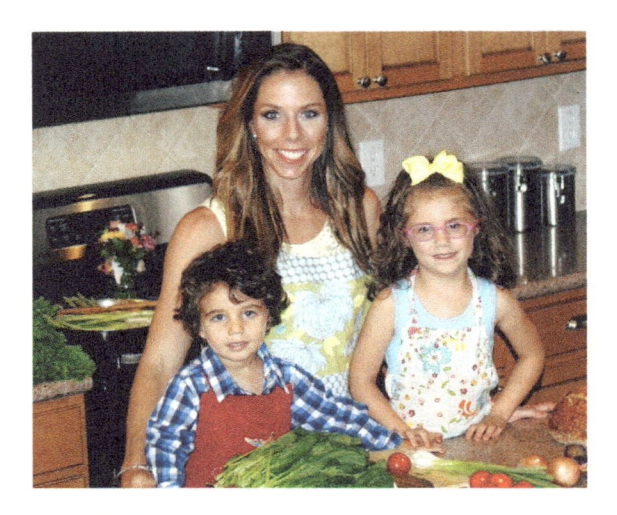

Nicole Eichinger with her kids Emma and Ethan.
This picture was the very first photo shoot for Nutrition's My Life, LLC!

Soon I knew, after a few things I saw at work and after my health began declining, that I wanted to work for myself. That is when I started Nutrition's My Life, LLC.

Nutrition's My Life was originally a way to help moms with their picky eaters. However, the more I went into my health journey and started to see improvements, the more I knew I needed to combine my nutrition degree and my personal experience as a health warrior to help other's struggling through the same thing.

That's when Nutrition's My Life, LLC became known for thyroid health!!

My Thyroid Story

Around this time my migraines were horrible, I didn't mention previously that migraines were something that started for me when I was in middle school. Migraines tend to plague the women in my family, especially under stressful times. And, at this time in my life, I had new mom problems meaning, I wasn't sleeping much with both a toddler and an infant.

 I was getting headaches daily. Three to four times a month I'd get a migraine that would wipe me out for the entire day, plus leave me with a migraine hangover the day after. It was horrible and I was desperate for help! I started seeing a Neurologist.

She had me try some medications when the migraines hit, but they would just put me to sleep and I would wake up still in pain. It didn't take the pain away and I couldn't be asleep all the tie, being mom. My migraines became so bad that I started developing an aura in my right eye. I would see a diamond in my vision and couldn't see through it. It was horrible.

My Thyroid Story

My neurologist had me undergo a sleep-deprived EEG, where I could only sleep 4 hours and then had to drive to the hospital to be hooked up to a monitor.

The nurses flashed strobe lights and different patterns/colors to see if they could induce a seizure. They failed at inducing a seizure however were successful at catching a migraine. *Another emotional and physical stress*!

Now flashing lights are something I'm working through, as they trigger my anxiety.

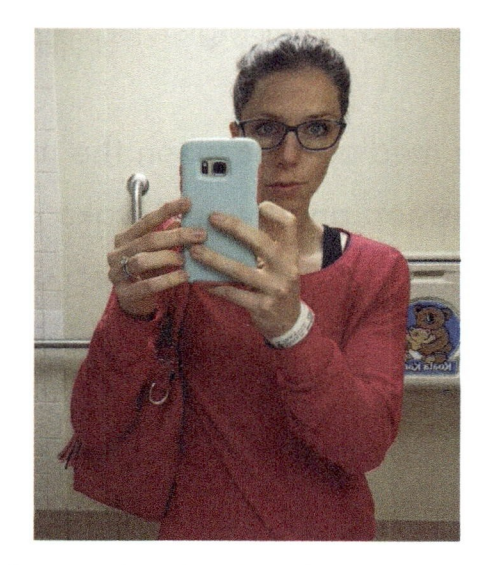

This picture is of me right after I had my sleep deprived EEG.

My Thyroid Story

I went back to my doctor for the results and she just told me to take three different kinds of medications. I told her I didn't want to do anymore meds, but I was curious about getting a piercing in my ear to help with the migraines. She laughed and told me it wouldn't work. I received a letter in the mail the following week that she was no longer going to be my doctor.

My long-term emotional and physical stress was taking their toll on my health.

I became a mean mom, you know the "get angry and snap at the kids" kind. I became someone who was miserable and my husband told me one day, "I don't even recognize you anymore. You're not the same woman I married." This made my heart break.

That's when I knew something had to change. I had to take back my health, and I started focusing on my migraines because it was the most painful thing at the time. Although I was working on my health, I still felt like my body was breaking down on me, literally! I would come home from work and collapse on the kitchen floor. Diaper bags, lunch box, purse, and the kids right there with me. I was running on empty but kept up the facade that I could do it all, that "I was ok."

My Thyroid Story

I really wasn't okay at all. I started having panic attacks. Full blown panic attacks and they were scary! My heart started to do funky things on me. I remember one time, on the way to see Santa with the kids in the back of the car, the scariest panic attack of my life happened! Luckily my husband was driving because I thought I was having a heart attack. I felt like there was a sheet of metal stuck through my chest, heavy and not bending as I tried to breathe.

I was always so tired; I ran off two to three cups of coffee a day. I felt like I had to prove something to someone... like I was trying to earn a mom of the year award, but foolish me, there was no award and no competition.

I eventually realized that coffee needed to go to help ease the mood swings, panic attacks, and massive migraines.

I abstained from all forms of caffeine for three months. No coffee, tea, or even chocolate. I gave my body the time to reset itself. It was hard at first and I did have some rebound headaches but I got through it. I found myself sleeping a bit more and the migraines subsiding a little without the constant caffeine.

My Thyroid Story

However, when you're sick, it's hard getting out of the "I'm sick mindset."

After improving my migraines, a new focus came to me... my heart! I saw a cardiologist because I was worried that I had a heart issue. I wore a heart monitor for a month, and I had a scope down my throat to look at my heart. I ended up waking up in the middle of having that tube down my throat which triggered a panic attack. *Even more emotional stress.*

I even did a stress test at the cardiologist! After all that, they found I do have something abnormal, but it only bothers me when I'm anxious or when my heart rate is up. I found that what I was feeling was just my anxiety and irregular heart beats caused by my thyroid hormone replacement meds.

I was under a lot of stress with my health and was wearing so many hats in my personal and work life (as I was still working part time for someone else and working part time for myself at Nutrition's My Life). I finally had to decide to quit my job at the dialysis clinic and work full time for myself.

My Thyroid Story

This was the best decision for my family and myself at the time. I had to take something off my plate so my body could start to heal and repair itself.

I started meditating in the mornings since I didn't have to rush to get off to work. I started gardening again and spending more time outside. I started using essential oils and paying more attention to chemicals in my food and environment. I was able to fully dive into my health journey.

I started researching more about migraines, anxiety, and thyroid disorders. I realized that if I provided just a little more nutrition to support these issues that I could go days without a headache and have more energy than I had in a long time. It wasn't as if I was eating bad before all this health journey started; I just wasn't meeting my nutrient demands. I had built a good foundation but needed more. I needed more.

I needed more healthy fats, more antioxidants, more B vitamins, more magnesium, more probiotics, more sleep, and more tools to help me heal.

My Thyroid Story

I started slowly adding in my tools that helped me feel my best. I started calling these tools my non-negotiables because I was tired of negotiating at the sake of my health, not anymore!

To be completely transparent, this has been a long process. I found little things like setting reminders in my phone to go off at crucial moments during the day when I knew I needed it the most, made a huge impact. Some of these reminders are to drink more water, to walk the dog, or to remind myself that I am loved!! I put sticky notes on my mirror and, moved my supplements out of my medicine cabinet into the kitchen where I knew I'd take them. I made things easier for myself and I learned to set boundaries.

I saw improvements, for sure, with all the new tools I was using. At the same time was still having heart palpitations, bone pain, and exhaustion from being on too much thyroid medication. My doctor kept saying I was in the "optimal" range, but my body was telling me something was wrong!

My Thyroid Story

Under the supervision of my endocrinologist, I was able to wean off my thyroid medication by slowly adding most of the tools you will find in this guide. And, to this day, I still have optimal level thyroid labs. Now did my endocrinologist believe it would work? Nope. He told me I'd be back in three months with weight gain. The doctor who put me on thyroid medication told me I'd have a set metabolism for life... I wonder why they only focused on my weight and not my actual symptoms?

I'm not cured of my ailments, but they're hanging in the background. They are not a bother to me most days. I occasionally have a migraine, I occasionally have a day where I need to rest more, and I occasionally can't sleep well. But, for the most part, I'm leaps and bounds above where I used to be.

I'm able to go on hikes, I'm able to rollerblade, I'm able to play tennis with my family on the weekends and attempt basketball with them (I'm just way better at soccer, lol). I'm able to ride my bike for hours. I'm able to garden and go to the beach with my family. I'm able to be active the way I want to be, and half of my thyroid is able to handle this without medication because of the tools you're going to learn in the coming chapters.

My Thyroid Story

Throughout this health guide, you're going to learn why it's so important to destress (not just keep pushing through like I did for so many years). You're going to understand why I store things in glass as much as I can. I'll share how the thyroid works, what foods support a healthy thyroid, and recipes that make it easy to eat those foods. We'll go into the supplements for a healthy thyroid and some other lifestyle components.

This is your all inclusive guide for everything thyroid health. This information may be beneficial if you have your full thyroid, no thyroid, or are a halfy like me! I'm excited for you to learn what your body and thyroid need!!

Remember, healing happens with consistency and time.
You got this!!

Nicole

Chapter One

Get to know the thyroid and the different thyroid disorders.

What is the Thyroid's Job?

I'm a big believer in being your own advocate for your health however, the body is complex and not enough education is done once someone is diagnosed with certain health conditions. This makes it difficult to advocate for yourself when the full picture isn't presented.

I was told, "Nicole, you are hypothyroid now that you have half a thyroid but don't worry, take this medication daily and you'll have a set metabolism for life!" That's why it took me so many years to finally figure out what my body needed to repair and heal.

I remember asking my endocrinologist after I had successfully come off thyroid medication if he was in need of a dietitian for his thyroid patients. He said he already had a dietitian on staff, but when I asked if the dietitian saw thyroid patients he said, "I've only sent diabetics to her, there's not much you can do with diet for a thyroid."

I've heard many other similar scary stories from my clients. I've heard, "I was told to do keto by my doctor, and I felt so much worse." Someone else told me their doctor recommended anti-anxiety medication because their labs were optimal. Unfortunately, many people are often misdiagnosed with anxiety or depression, when, in reality, it's the thyroid's doing! I'm excited to help give you the knowledge to understand your body and thyroid condition better.

What is the Thyroid's Job?

The thyroid is a butterfly-shaped gland that is responsible for the metabolism of almost every cell in your body. This means improving thyroid health requires focusing on more than just the thyroid gland.

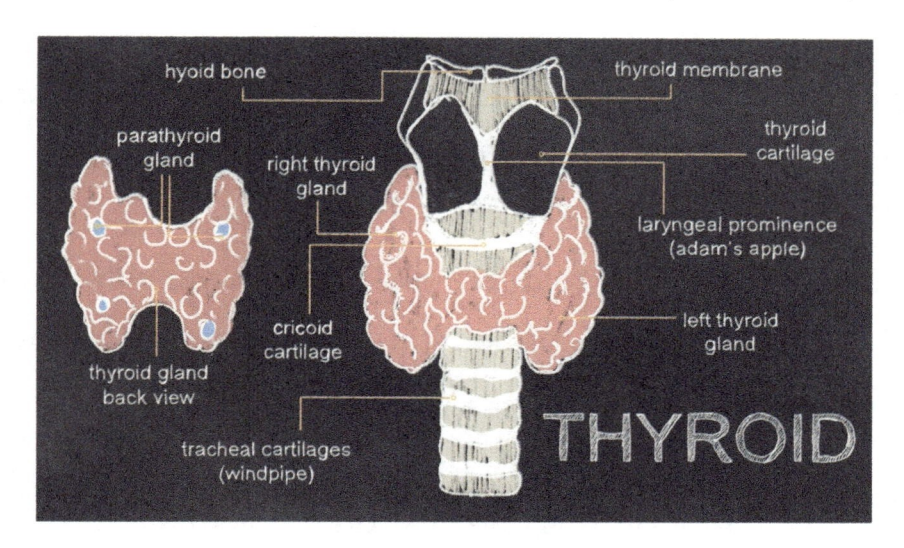

The thyroid's hormones regulate vital body functions, including:
- Breathing
- Heart rate
- Central and peripheral nervous systems
- Body weight
- Muscle strength
- Menstrual cycles
- Body temperature
- Cholesterol levels
- Metabolic Rate
- & so much more!

How Does The Thyroid Work?

Making active thyroid hormones starts in the brain. The hypothalamus produces a hormone called thyrotropin-releasing hormone, TRH.

TRH stimulates the pituitary gland to make the hormone most people are familiar with, thyroid stimulating hormone or TSH.

TSH then stimulates the thyroid to make the other thyroid hormones, T4 and T3. In fact, over 90% of hormones produced in the thyroid are inactive T4.

T4 relies on two major organs, the liver and digestive tract, to be converted into the active thyroid hormone, T3. These two organs are crucial for optimal thyroid health and will be discussed on the next few pages in depth.

Even if you don't have a thyroid, you have a way to impact your thyroid health if you optimize these two important thyroid-supporting organs.

How Does the Thyroid Work?

Liver

The liver plays a crucial role in thyroid health.

More T4 to T3 conversion occurs in the liver than anywhere else in the body. A complex relationship exists between the thyroid gland and the liver in both health and disease (1). This is where the essential nutrients for thyroid health come into play and why it's important to incorporate foods that support those nutrients daily. More on these nutrients in chapter seven.

When there is liver damage present, the thyroid is negatively affected. Focusing on liver health can be beneficial for improved thyroid levels and symptoms. To understand how to improve liver health, we have to first determine the cause. Unstable blood glucose levels, a diet rich in saturated fats (animal products or fried foods), and obesity are the most common causes of liver damage that I have seen in my career as a registered dietitian.

How Does The Thyroid Work?

Liver

If you're the type of person that eats a steak the size of their head, eats fast food at most meals, skips breakfast often, and/or drinks a lot of alcohol, you might be at a higher risk of having liver damage. Initially you may start to see elevated liver enzymes and triglycerides.

However, if poor eating and lifestyle habits continue, liver damage will progress. I see it happen in my practice. Liver damage in the early stages - fatty liver disease - is more common than you may think. Especially in those with insulin resistance. Luckily reversing early stage liver damage is doable with diet and lifestyle changes.

The liver has over 500 vital roles in the body an one of them is the conversion of T4 to T3. Fortunately, many of the anti-inflammatory foods discussed in this book also support the liver.

One thing that's been shown to help with improving liver health is increasing plant intake while decreasing animal sources of protein. I'm not saying you have to omit all animal sources, but reflect on your intake and follow the plate method discussed later in this book.

How Does the Thyroid Work?

Liver

The benefits of eating more plants for liver health comes from a kind of amino acids found in plants. Amino acids are the building blocks of proteins and the types of amino acids found in plants are called branch chain amino acids, BCAAs. People with liver disease tend to have low levels of BCAAs and can develop something called, cachexia or muscle wasting.

The cool thing about focusing on BCAAs is that these foods also contain antioxidants. I like to think of antioxidants as the plant's superpowers! Plants have protective properties like antioxidants, polyphenols and flavonoids. When we eat plants, those protective properties work inside our bodies to protect us from harmful substances.

Every color of fruits and vegetables provides a different antioxidant. This is why "eating the rainbow" is so helpful! Aim to eat a variety of colors at every meal and you'll automatically eat foods that contain a variety of these protective properties!!

How Does The Thyroid Work?

Liver Supporting Tips:

- Use the plate method for more plants and less meat (see chapter nine).
- Incorporate foods rich in antioxidants- specifically glutathione. Glutathione plays crucial roles in the detoxification and antioxidant systems of cells (2).
  - Beets, spinach, & blueberries are my top favorite antioxidant and glutathione rich foods.
- Consistently eat throughout the day to help stabilize blood sugars.
- More water, less alcohol.

Dietitian Pro Tips:

- Set reminders on your phone to drink water.
- Choose a large water bottle with a straw.
- Meal prep or double a dinner recipe, so you can have lunches prepared for the next day.
- Try to eat the rainbow at every meal.

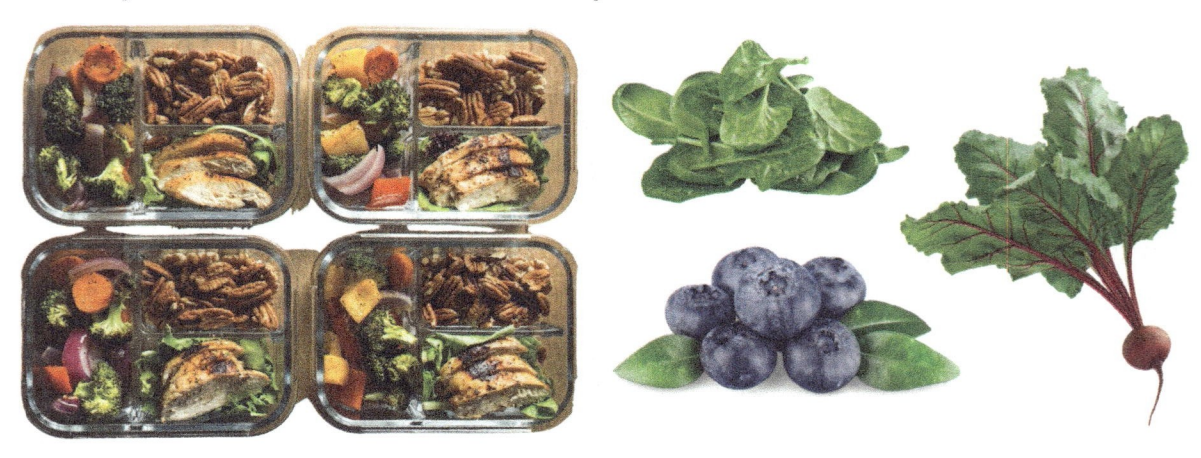

How Does The Thyroid Work?

Digestion

20 - 30% of the conversion of T4 to T3 occurs within the digestive lining.

Improving your digestive tract health can benefit you in many ways. It actually helps you absorb your nutrition better, decrease your risk of autoimmunity (that is to say, if you have an autoimmune disease it may help it improve, or if you don't have one, it may decrease your risk of developing one), decreases inflammation, improves hormone levels, improves cholesterol levels, may decrease anxiety and stress, and can even lead to weight loss.

The digestive tract is very complex, but to simplify it for you, there are two major structures: small intestine and large intestine. The large intestine is supposed to house between five to seven pounds of healthy bacteria in an adult person. Healthy bacteria, or probiotics, are necessary for our health.

Probiotics digest fiber in the foods we eat and in return provide our digestive tract (gut wall) with fuel. This is how the body repairs the gut wall lining which is crucial for nutrient absorption, lowering inflammation, reducing stress, and of course hormone health.

How Does the Thyroid Work?

Gut Health 101

1. Prebiotic containing foods like leeks, oats, onions, garlic, asparagus, and beans are fuel for the live bacteria, probiotics.

2. Probiotics like kombucha, yogurt, miso, fermented cabbage, and probiotic supplements contain the live, beneficial bacteria that eat fiber in the foods we consume.

3. Drink enough water throughout the day to help with digestion. Lack of water can lead to constipation.

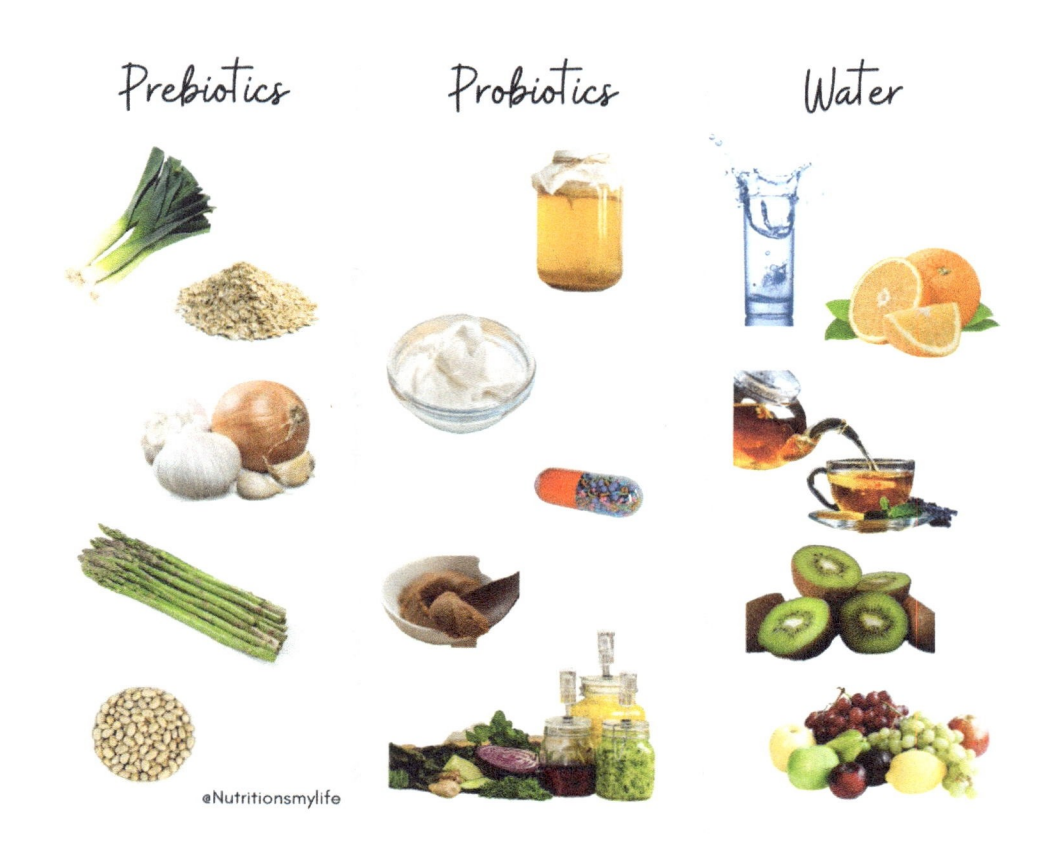

Prebiotics *Probiotics* *Water*

@Nutritionsmylife

How Does the Thyroid Work?

Digestion and Stress

One thing that gets overlooked in digestive health is the overall state of the body. What I mean is, "are you stressed or calm while you're eating?" Blood flow is shunted away from the intestines when in a state of stress, anxiety, or worry. This happens for our survival.

If you saw a bear on a hike, your body would go into fight or flight mode. Fight or flight mode is also called the sympathetic nervous system. During fight or flight the body is in survival mode, and ready to fight or run away. The blood gets shunted away from the intestines and goes to the muscles to help you fight or flee the scene.

Take notice of the state your body is in before you eat if you've been experiencing bloating, pain, diarrhea, or constipation. Many of my clients that have digestive issues love this part of the repairing of gut health because it has a bigger impact than you might think.

I may sound like a broken record throughout the book as I remind you to stress less. However, stress is like a thief in the night. It's going to leave you feeling like you have nothing left, it's going to make you feel uncomfortable, and it's going to make you feel frustrated.

How Does The Thyroid Work?

Digestion and Stress

If you are stressed and it's time to eat, try one or more of these stress reduction tools to help you digest and absorb your nutrition better.

1. Take deep belly breathes. Many people who are stressed or anxious take short shallow breathes. Sit or stand up straight. Place your hands on your stomach and take a deep belly breath. You should feel your hands move away from each other.
2. Try box breathing, also known as square breathing. Box breathing is something used by the military and it's really quite simple. Find a window, door, or square of some sort to look at. Start on the bottom left side, take a deep breath for four seconds while tracing your eyes up to the top left corner. Hold the inhale for four seconds as you move horizontally to the right top corner. Once your eyes reach the top right corner, exhale for four seconds as you move to the bottom right corner. Once your eyes hit the bottom right corner, hold the exhaled out breath for four seconds.
3. A quick dance party can do wonders to get you out of a funk.
4. Go outside, take a deep breathe, and tell yourself five things you're grateful for that you can see, smell, or hear around you.
5. Take a short and easy walk.
6. Plan ahead so you have time to eat before rushing out the door. Never eat while rushing.

How Does the Thyroid Work?

Slow digestion and Serotonin

Motility refers to the movement of food through the intestines. This movement is called peristalsis. With hypothyroidism, many people end up being constipated due to the slow metabolism and subsequently, slow motility. This can contribute to the bloating and discomfort that many people experience with hypothyroidism.

Improving the thyroid will help improve motility but doing things like lowering stress while eating, repairing the gut wall with probiotics, and eating foods rich in fiber, will help you feel better in more ways than just physically. Try to incorporate more of the foods on the gut friendly food list, found in three pages, to aid in digestion.

Did you know that there is a gut brain connection?

The vagus nerve connects the digestive tract to the brain. This means our gut hears what we are thinking. The other way it's connected is through serotonin. Serotonin is the feel-good hormone and up to 95% of it is made in the digestive tract.

How Does the Thyroid Work?

Slow digestion and Serotonin

Gut bacteria produce hundreds of neurochemicals that the brain uses to regulate basic physiological processes as well as mental processes such as learning, memory and mood. For example, gut bacteria manufacture about 95% of the body's supply of serotonin, which influences both mood and GI activity (3).

This is why it's so important to focus on gut health repair and mindset at the same time. I believe so strongly that the body will not heal without working on your mindset that I created an online course focused on helping people repair their digestion. This course is called Mind Your Gut and is available on my website, www.nutritionsmylife.com.

For serotonin to be made, gut bacteria needs to metabolize the precursor of serotonin, tryptophan. Tryptophan is an amino acid that's abundant in beef, salmon, pumpkin seeds, oatmeal and eggs.

Digestive health, just like thyroid health, is complex. On the next page, you'll find simplified steps for optimal gut health and on the following page you'll find the gut friendly food list.

How Does The Thyroid Work?

Digestion Non-Negotiables

Digestive health is so important and has such a big impact on our health, that I've made the following non-negotiables.

1 Check in with yourself before eating. Remember that eating while stress is just having expensive poop, you're not going to absorb much nutrition from the food.

2 Probiotics are the beneficial bacteria that need to be replenished daily by eating fermented food and/or taking probiotic supplementation. After beneficial probiotics eat fiber, they make fuel for the gut wall called short chain fatty acids. Probiotics are also in charge of helping tryptophan turn into serotonin.

3 Eat a diet rich in prebiotics. Prebiotics are a type of dietary fiber that fuel the beneficial bacteria in the digestive tract. This helps digest our food and also helps with other processes in the body.

4 Adequate water intake is necessary for a healthy digestive environment. Not enough water may lead to constipation.

Healthy Thyroid Guide

Gut Friendly Foods

Foods that Reduce Inflammation

Omega 3 Fatty Acids

- Walnuts
- Cashews
- Brazil Nuts
- Avocado
- Olives
- Milled Flaxseed
- Salmon
- Anchovies

Antioxidants

- Blueberries
- Cherries
- Cranberries
- Sweet Potato
- Spinach & Kale
- Red Cabbage
- Beets
- Beans & legumes
- Broccoli

Spices & Herbs

- Turmeric
- Ginger
- Cinnamon
- Cardamom
- Oregano
- Cilantro
- Basil
- Parsley
- Fennel

Prebiotic Foods

Foods that the live bacteria in your gut eat.

- Onion
- Garlic
- Leeks
- Soybeans
- Resistant Starch (oats, cooled rice, whole grains, legumes, beans, green bananas)

Probiotic Foods

Live bacteria containing foods

- Kimchi
- Kombucha
- Miso
- Suerkraut
- Keifer
- Non-Dairy Yogurts

Supplements that support a healthy gut.

- L-Glutamine
- Probiotics
- Peppermint Tea
- Chamomile Tea
- Marshmallow Root
- Colostrum
- Magnesium or Dandelion for constipation
- Reishi, Chaga & Maitake medicinal mushrooms

Chapter Two

Different Thyroid Disorders

Different Thyroid Disorders

As you noticed in chapter one, the thyroid controls a lot of the daily functions of the body. It's easy to see why so many people struggle with their thyroid health because it can be confused with other issues.

Here is what I mean, if you've had menstrual cycle issues and you go see your gynecologist (gyno), your gyno might put you on birth control. You might see your primary care physician to discuss weight gain and being tired, classic signs of hypothyroidism. However, many people are given a prescription for an anti-depressant, as those are also classic signs of depression. Then what tends to happen is the hypothyroidism is left untreated becomes worse months or years later.

It infuriates me that this is how our healthcare system tends to be, a revolving door of patients. I've worked in hospitals and clinics where we had to submit our productivity to the managers, which showed how many patients I saw in a day. I was told by a manager once, "your pumping is getting in the way of your productivity." Mind you, I would do my calculations for the 18 - 21 different neonatal intensive care infants I had to see during my shift, and still fit my pumping in. This pressure from healthcare management is why I started my own business, and this furry is a big reason why I wrote this book for you.

On the next few pages, you'll start to understand the differences between the thyroid disorders and causes behind them. Hopefully this will help you navigate the symptoms of thyroid issues better.
The thyroid disorders are: Hypothyroidism, Hashimoto's Thyroiditis (autoimmune), Hyperthyroidism, Graves' Disease (autoimmune), and thyroid cancer.

Different Thyroid Disorders

Hypothyroid

The mayo clinic defines hypothyroidism (underactive thyroid) as a condition in which your thyroid gland doesn't produce enough of certain crucial hormones (4).

Hypothyroidism can be triggered by multiple issues. For me, it was caused by the removal of half my thyroid due to radiation exposure from a severe non-healing spiral fracture to my right humerus. For others, it may be trauma or stress related (i.e. childbirth, divorce, death in the family, etc.), an iodine deficiency, medications such as lithium for a psychiatric disorder, surgical removal of the thyroid, or an autoimmune response (4).

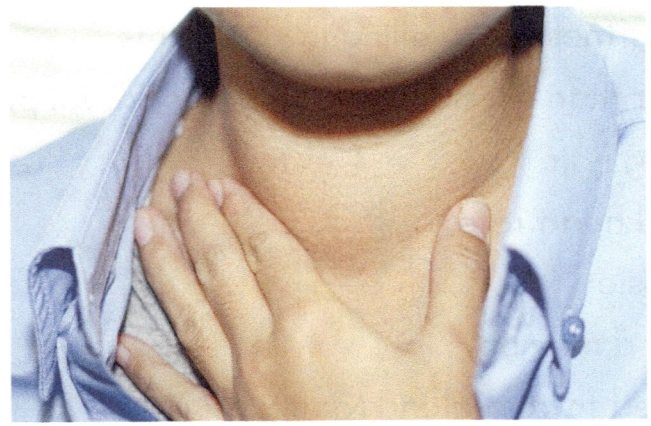

Goiter

Different Thyroid Disorders

Hypothyroid

Hypothyroidism signs and symptoms may include:

- Fatigue
- Increased sensitivity to cold
- Constipation
- Dry skin
- Weight gain
- Puffy face
- Hoarseness
- Muscle weakness
- Elevated blood cholesterol level
- Muscle aches, tenderness and stiffness
- Pain, stiffness or swelling in your joints
- Heavier than normal or irregular menstrual periods
- Thinning hair
- Slowed heart rate
- Depression
- Impaired memory
- Enlarged thyroid gland (goiter)

Different Thyroid Disorders

Thyroid symptoms can be improved with nutrition and lifestyle changes. However, this does not guarantee you will be cured with nutrition and lifestyle changes alone. It all depends on whether your body's nutrient demands are met and if the body is in the right environment (less stress, happy, sleeping well, etc.) to heal.

The body is designed to heal itself, but some people need a little more help than others. Some people are born with inborn errors, no fault of their own, it just happens. Take me for example, I'm unable to convert my B vitamins into their active form. It is a genetic mutation, called MTHFR, that occurs more frequently in people of European descent. MTHFR stands for Methylenetetrahydrofolate reductase. Taking methylated B vitamins in a supplement is how to help someone's body with MTHFR have a properly functioning nervous system and proper production of red blood cells, which could both suffer if low in B vitamins.

Another example are autoimmune disorders. Autoimmune disorders cause the body to lack the tools to work properly like in Hashimoto's disease. With Hashimoto's disease the body is essentially attacking its own thyroid gland, causing improper thyroid hormone amounts to be made. If we give the body the tools to protect the thyroid, reduce risk of autoimmunity through gut health repair, and promote stress and inflammation reduction, then the body is able to function properly.

Different Thyroid Disorders

Hypothyroid

Having anxiety, depression, or stress are other examples of how the body wants to heal but needs more help. Anxiety, for example, increases the demand of B vitamins, magnesium, and healthy fats.

If you're not meeting those demands, you might still feel fatigued and anxious. You may even be eating foods that contain B vitamins, magnesium and healthy fats but it may not be enough for the amount you're burning through!

I've had people tell me they're eating healthy fats, but when I go through their day to see what they're eating, it's very minimal to what their body is needing. I'll see people eat salmon at dinner one day and then add nuts the next day to help with their health fat intake. However, someone with higher nutrient demands needs to add a source at every meal, plus snacks, to get close to what their body requires. Their intake is only once a day for healthy fats, versus the actual demand of three to four times a day.

The body wants to repair itself we just have to provide it the tools.

Different Thyroid Disorders

Hypothyroid

It's important to understand that even if your thyroid has been surgically removed, the tools in this healthy thyroid guide can help! Hypothyroidism can be improved with or without thyroid supplemental medication.

Hypothyroidism takes time to heal; I like to tell my clients that you can improve your thyroid's health and/or your body's health but it doesn't mean you get to be carefree for the rest of your life. The thyroid is influenced by so many things, which means a healthy thyroid only happens with a life-long commitment to a healthy lifestyle!

This is why one of my favorite sayings is "count your chemicals, not your calories". It helps you put the focus on quality, because quality matters!

In my opinion, the best thing for someone who has hypothyroidism (or any health struggle) to do is find ways to navigate stress and anxiety. Stress and anxiety really are major culprits to people's health. Your body remembers how to return to unhealthy.

Different Thyroid Disorders

Hashimoto's Thyroiditis: Autoimmune

Many of my thyroid clients have weight loss as their major goal, but as they travel down that path they learn to listen to how their body is changing and improving. They accomplish their weight loss and are overall healthier by getting back into tune with themselves.

Meditation or gratitude practices are important for stress reduction, as well as learning to listen to your body. Stress reduction is crucial for people with an autoimmune disorder. If you have yet to incorporate meditation or gratitude into your day...then here's your sign to start something! Both practices can help you reduce stress and bring you into the present moment. Many people with a thyroid disorder tend to be more stressed and have more anxiety. It's time to work on your mental health as well. I see a therapist once a month and highly recommend all my thyroid warriors to do the same.

Learning to be your own compass helps you navigate life. Some days you may need to rest more, honor yourself by resting. Some days you may feel like you can't do it, have a cry and feel through the emotions, don't sit and hold it in. I don't know how many time's I've heard, "I feel like I'm crazy" from different clients because of how complex the thyroid is and how difficult this journey can be.

Different Thyroid Disorders

Hashimoto's Thyroiditis: Autoimmune

Hashimoto's disease is a condition in which your immune system attacks your thyroid and is the most common cause of hypothyroidism (5). A doctor may diagnose Hashimoto's Thyroiditis when there are TPO antibodies present greater than 9 IU/mL. Symptoms of Hashimoto's are the ones listed in hypothyroid section five pages ago, because having Hashimoto's also means you're hypothyroid.

I have seen women with normal TSH levels get told for years their labs are fine despite feeling extreme fatigue. Then, they go see a different doctor that's willing to test TPO Antibodies and they're typically in the thousands range (one recently was 1,500! It's supposed to be less than 9!!)

Always remember, your symptoms are telling you something. The good part of your healthy thyroid journey is that the best indicator that what you're doing is working comes from asking yourself,
"HOW AM I FEELING?!!"

I cannot stress enough how important it is to check in with yourself.

Different Thyroid Disorders

Hashimoto's Thyroiditis: Autoimmune

Many of my thyroid clients have weight loss as their major goal, but as they travel down that path they learn to listen to how their body is changing and improving. They accomplish their weight loss and are overall healthier by getting back into tune with themselves.

Meditation or gratitude practices are important for stress reduction, as well as learning to listen to your body. Stress reduction is crucial for people with an autoimmune disorder. If you have yet to incorporate meditation or gratitude into your day...then here's your sign to start something! Both practices can help you reduce stress and bring you into the present moment. Many people with a thyroid disorder tend to be more stressed and have more anxiety. It's time to work on your mental health as well. I see a therapist once a month and highly recommend all my thyroid warriors to do the same.

Learning to be your own compass helps you navigate life. Some days you may need to rest more, honor yourself by resting. Some days you may feel like you can't do it, have a cry and feel through the emotions, don't sit and hold it in. I don't know how many time's I've heard, "I feel like I'm crazy" from different clients because of how complex the thyroid is and how difficult this journey can be.

Different Thyroid Disorders

Hashimoto's Thyroiditis: Autoimmune

I remember feeling very lonely at the beginning of my health journey, but I reminded my self I just had to try my best and if my best that day was only to take a nap to recharge then that's ok. But I learned not to let those days become me!

I have seen many people with Hashimoto's also have another autoimmune disorder. If you are someone who has multiple autoimmune disorders, many times we can focus on the same things to help improve them all. I find that improving gut health, inflammation, and stress helps improve autoimmune symptoms across the board. A diet high in antioxidants (like the Selenium containing ones listed in chapter seven) is really helpful in protecting the body. Antioxidants are in the colors of foods. Start incorporating more fruits and vegetables of many colors #eattherainbow. Many of the tools in this book are helpful for reducing all types of autoimmunity.

I know many people who have been told that medication is the only way to live a "normal" life with an autoimmune disorder. I find this so frustrating. I have seen people's TPO go from 2000 down to 20 by eating a diet rich in anti-inflammatory foods and by living a healthy lifestyle. You'll learn more about the lifestyle factors in chapter four.

Again, the body wants to repair itself, we just have to provide it the tools.

Different Thyroid Disorders

The photo, pictured below, was a stock photo that was suggested for me to use while making this guide and it shocked me with all the medications. It's sad because many people are placed on anti-anxiety meds, anti-depressants, and even cholesterol medications in addition to their thyroid meds.

But if they just optimize their thyroid health, like outlined in this book, then those mental health meds won't always be necessary. I'm not saying they don't have their time and place, because they do, but it's not the only solution. This is not me saying to stop your medication either, see your doctor.

In general, I see mental health medications prescribed first, before the thyroid is addressed. I was on anti-anxiety and anti-depressants before I started my thyroid replacement therapy. Now I speak with a therapist once a month instead of taking anti-anxiety or depression medication. Now I use lifestyle habits and eat to support my body instead of taking thyroid medication. I'm not promising miracles with this book, but I am giving you options.

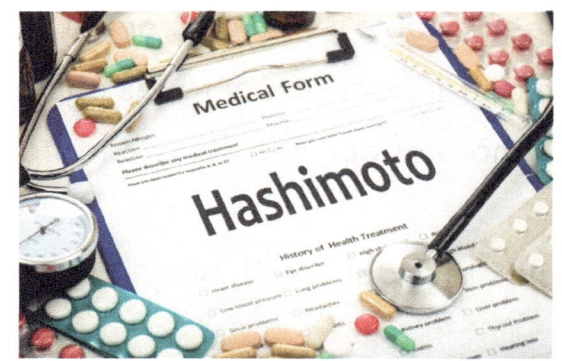

Different Thyroid Disorders

Hashimoto's Thyroiditis: Autoimmune

Just because you have an autoimmune disease, does not mean you can't be in control of your health. That doctor saying, "This pill is your set metabolism for life," (yes that is exactly what my original thyroid medication prescribing doctor told me) is not actually 100% knowledgeable on thyroid health. Not all doctors are well versed in the thyroid world, and I have seen many doctors just prescribe thyroid medication without any other intervention.

When it comes to an autoimmune disorder, gut health is a major focus. I have seen it over and over again, thyroid labs improve when we focus on improving digestive health by; reducing stress and inflammation while increasing nutrient-dense foods.

Know that improving your autoimmune disorder is a lifelong commitment. Once you improve your health, you have to keep using the tools that got you there. If you don't, you'll end back up in old habits and routines, which will likely result in an increase in autoimmunity. Lifestyle changes for the better is how we support the goals we have for our body.

Different Thyroid Disorders

Hyperthyroid:
Hyperthyroidism (overactive thyroid) occurs when your thyroid gland produces too much of the hormone thyroxine. Hyperthyroidism can accelerate your body's metabolism, causing unintentional weight loss and a rapid or irregular heartbeat.

Some people with Hashimoto's disease will swing between hypothyroid and hyperthyroid. This typically occurs during a time of stress (and/or requires gut health repair.)

Graves Disease: Graves' disease is an immune system disorder that results in the overproduction of thyroid hormones (hyperthyroidism) (6).

Common signs and symptoms of Graves' disease include:
- Anxiety and irritability
- A fine tremor of the hands or fingers
- Heat sensitivity and an increase in perspiration or warm, moist skin
- Weight loss, despite normal eating habits
- Enlargement of the thyroid gland (goiter)
- Change in menstrual cycles
- Erectile dysfunction or reduced libido
- Frequent bowel movements
- Bulging eyes (Graves' ophthalmopathy)
- Fatigue
- Thick, red skin usually on the shins or tops of the feet (Graves' dermopathy)
- Rapid or irregular heartbeat (palpitations)
- Sleep disturbance

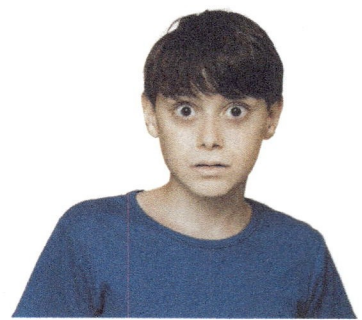

Bulging eyes

Different Thyroid Disorders

Many people with hyperthyroidism will undergo radioactive iodine treatment. Radioactive iodine is taken up by the thyroid, and destroys the cells in the thyroid gland. This has the effect of reducing the amount of thyroxine made by the thyroid gland and may also reduce the size of the gland.

This may affect both men and women's reproductive hormones short term but they tend to normalize out. It's important to see your doctor regularly as hyperthyroidism can lead to serious health issues.

*The optimal health plan for hyperthyroidism should be the same as what you find in this guide except for the need to decrease intake of **tyrosine and iodine rich foods.** Tyrosine and iodine encourage production of T4 and T3 which we want reduced. These foods are found in chapter seven.

Weight Gain: Many people struggle to gain weight when in a state of hyperthyroidism. A diet that includes healthy fat options at every meal and snack is beneficial for providing extra calories, but it also helps reduce any inflammation and helps with the nervous system. I recommend this for most people anyway. I encourage a thumb's worth of healthy fat every meal; however people with hyperthyroidism may need double this. This is not me saying to just double up on fish oil, it's best to incorporate a variety in your meals. Try to include avocados, nuts, seeds, olives, olive oil, fatty fish, and grass-fed beef.

Different Thyroid Disorders

Thyroid Cancer

I was lucky to catch my thyroid when I did, as the doctor told me it would have turned into cancer. According to cancer.gov, there are four main types of thyroid cancer. These are papillary, follicular, medullary, and anaplastic. Papillary is see most often in people with thyroid cancer.

Many people start with a lump in their throat, myself included. You'll likely receive bloodwork and a thyroid biopsy. The biopsy is nothing to be scared about but it's not pleasant feeling a needle inside your throat. I was a bit sore after mine however it didn't last for long. Your doctor will be able to give you a treatment plan.

In cancer, nutrition plays a crucial role. Many of my patients in the past found making shakes very helpful. When making a shake think about making it a complete meal with protein powder or nut/seed butters, yogurt, vegetables (frozen cauliflower & spinach blend up nicely), fruit, a source of healthy fats (fish oil, milled flaxseed, or chia seeds), and liquid.

If you have half or all of your thyroid removed, you may be diagnosed with hypothyroidism by your physician. The contents in this book may be extremely beneficial.

Chapter Three

Thyroid Hormones and Labs

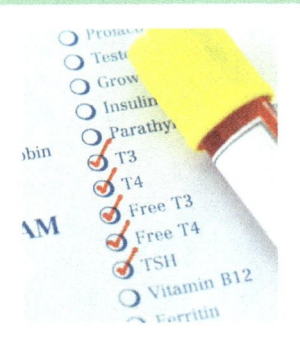

Thyroid Hormones

TSH is produced by the pituitary gland which is the signal for your thyroid to make T4 and T3 hormones.

All lab data from mayocliniclabs.com

TSH: Thyroid Stimulating Hormone
Adults: 0.3 - 4.2 mIU/L (optimal range is 0.3 - 2.5 mIU/L)
Too much: hypothyroid
Too little: hyperthyroid

TSH is a glycoprotein hormone (g*lyco means glucose, thus supporting need for carbohydrates in your diet*). The role of TSH is to stimulate the thyroid to make T4 and T3 hormones.

Free T4: Thyroxine
Adults: 0.9-1.7 ng/dL
Too much = hyperthyroid
Too little = hypothyroid

Inactive thyroid hormone and is produced in the thyroid gland. Needs to be converted into active T3.

Free T3: Triiodothyronine
> or =1 year: 2.8-4.4 pg/mL
Too much = hyperthyroid
Too little = hypothyroid

Most active thyroid hormone. Most conversion of T3 takes place in the liver.

Thyroid Hormones

All lab data from mayocliniclabs.com

TSH (Thyroid Stimulating Hormone)

Produced by pituitary gland. Tells your thyroid (which needs selenium foods) to make active thyroid hormones: T3 and T4

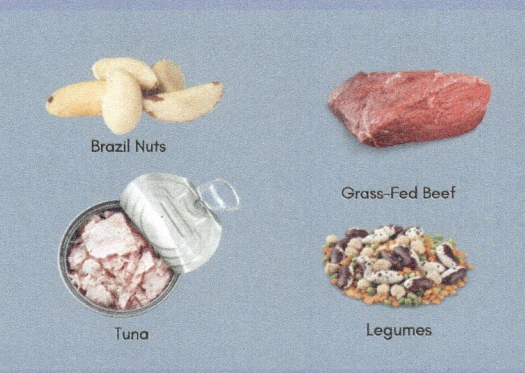

Selenium

- Brazil Nuts
- Grass-Fed Beef
- Tuna
- Legumes

↑ > 4.20 mIU/mL

Too Much = hypo

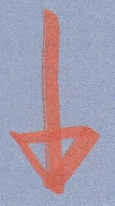

↓ < 0.30 – mIU/mL

Too little = hyper

T3 & T4 are made by the thyroid combining iodine & tyrosine.

Only 20% of thyroid hormones made from the thyroid itself is T3. The liver, digestive tract, and kidneys provide locations for the remainder of active T3 hormones to be converted from T4. Tyrosine and iodine are necessary for this to happen. See food sources below.

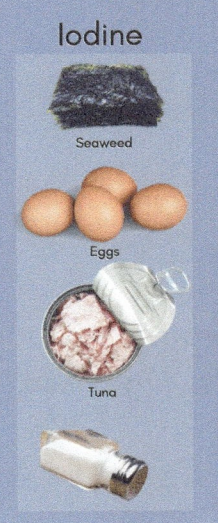

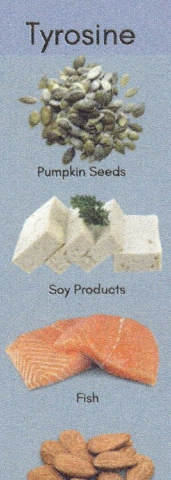

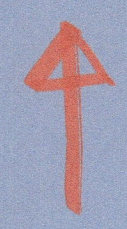

Iodine
- Seaweed
- Eggs
- Tuna

Tyrosine
- Pumpkin Seeds
- Soy Products
- Fish

↑ Too Much T4 & T3 = hyper

↓ Too little T4 & T3 = hypo

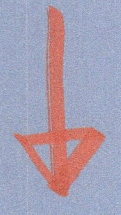

61

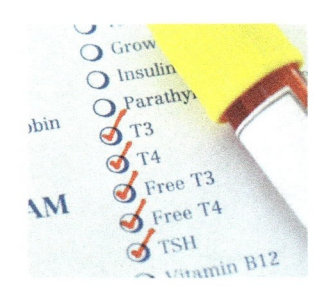

Thyroid Hormones

Understanding your thyroid hormones and labs are a great way to be empowered in your health!
All lab data from mayocliniclabs.com

rT3: Reverse T3

10 - 24 ng/dL
Has iodines in different locations atomically than T3 because the body sometimes prefers rT3 instead of T3.

High rT3 is typically caused by stress, trauma, decreased caloric intake (like in anorexia or while dieting), inflammation, toxins, liver dysfunction and medications.

TPO Antibodies: Thyroxine Peroxidase Antibodies

The measured serum level should be less than 9 IU/mL.
Testing TPO antibody levels provides the most sensitive test for detecting autoimmune thyroid disease. Thyroxine Peroxidase is actually an enzyme that helps make T4 and T3. The test that many people receive is measuring the antibodies against TPO.

TBG: Thyroxine Binding Globulin
Males: 12 - 26 mcg/mL
Females: 11 - 27 mcg/mL

Responsible for transporting T4 and T3 in the bloodstream.
Elevated TBG levels are associated with influences such as pregnancy, genetic predisposition, oral contraceptives, and estrogen therapy.
TBG levels can decrease with androgenic or anabolic steroids, large doses of glucocorticoids, liver disease, nephrotic syndrome, etc.

Know Your Labs

Below are some other supporting labs that may be beneficial in helping with understanding the thyroid levels. Not everyone needs every lab, so please see your dietitian or doctor for guidance.

If you want certain labs drawn-ask! You're paying for them, the doctor has no right to say no to supporting labs and if they do, you have the right to change doctors. Some lab drawing companies don't require doctor's orders. You may be able to order labs from home. Just know you have options. I've heard stories over the years and have first handed been told "that's an expensive lab." I say educate yourself for a reason. You have to be your own advocate!

All lab tests referenced from Mayo Clinic Laboratories

RBC: This test is a count of the actual number of red blood cells in your blood sample.

Hemoglobin: This measures the total amount of oxygen-carrying protein in the blood.

HCT: Hematocrit measures the percentage of your blood volume consisting of red blood cells.

MCV: Mean corpuscular volume is a measurement of the average size of your red blood cells. Small size can indicate iron deficiency anemia and too large can indicate pernicious anemia.

WBC: The test is a count of the number of white blood cells in your blood sample. White blood cells help protect against infections and also play a role in inflammation.

Know Your Labs

25(OH) Vitamin D:
< 30 nmol/L is considered deficient.
30 – < 50 is insufficient for bone and overall health.
> 50 is generally sufficient for most people. *(I like it in the 60 range)*
> 125 is linked to potential adverse effects.
This tells you the amount of 25-hydroxyvitamin D in your blood. It is a good indication of how much vitamin D your body has (7).

Cholesterol: The thyroid controls cholesterol's metabolism and has a positive correlation with TSH and Cholesterol.

HDL CHOLESTEROL: High Density Lipoprotein
Males > or = 40 mg/dL
Females > or = 50 mg/dL

LDL CHOLESTEROL: Low Density Lipoprotein
Adults: Desirable: < 100 mg/dL

Vitamin B12: Cobalamin.
Range: 180 – 914 ng/L
B12 is found in foods from animals, such as red meat, fish, poultry, milk, yogurt, and eggs. B12 is helpful in making proteins, energy production and can affect your blood cell size if you don't have enough. I notice my clients feel the best around the 800 – 900 range.

Know Your Labs

Folate (Vitamin B9) refers to a naturally occurring form of the vitamin, whereas folic acid refers to the supplement added to foods and drinks. Folate is found in leafy green vegetables, citrus fruits, dry beans and peas, liver, and yeast.

Selenium:
>1 year: 70 - 150 ng/mL
This is an essential element–it plays a role in thyroid health, immune health, and is a potent antioxidant.

Iodine:
Range: 40-92 ng/mL

Iodine is an essential element that is required for thyroid hormone production. The measurement of iodine serves as an index of adequate dietary iodine intake and iodine overload, particularly from iodine-containing drugs such as amiodarone.

HbA1c: Hemoglobin A1c
HbA1c Reference Range: 4.0 - 5.6%

The HbA1c level reflects the mean glucose concentration over the previous period (approximately 8 - 12 weeks, depending on the individual).

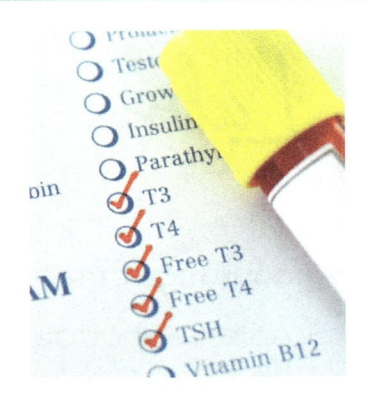

Speak Up

Be Your Own Advocate!!

Take questions or request for labs you'd like drawn with you on a piece of paper so you can remember to ask the doctor. Many people find it difficult to remember everything that was said in a doctor's visit, note taking can help!

Write notes down before the visit and then write down key words during your appointment, or have the doctor repeat what was said so you can write it down.

Confusion and being overwhelmed at a visit is a real thing.

Take control by first learning about your disorder/condition/health struggle and then asking questions. If the doctor is not willing to answer or give you what you need, it's ok to get a second opinion. If you have an insurance that requires a PCP, primary care physician, call the insurance company and have them assign you a new one.

Advocate for yourself because you deserve the best care!

Chapter Four

Lifestyle Factors that Influence the Thyroid

Lifestyle Factors
That Influence the Thyroid

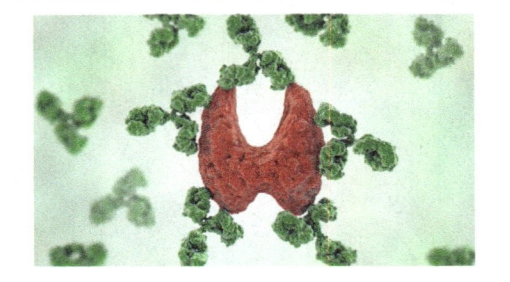

The thyroid influences almost every cell in the body and therefore is influenced by many factors itself. Don't underestimate the impact lifestyle factors can have on the thyroid and overall health.

I'm a great example of how focusing on lifestyle can have a big impact. Being a registered dietitian and feeding my body well wasn't enough, I still had many hypothyroid symptoms and many health problems. Things really changed for the better once I started focusing on my sleep, my mindset, learning how to stress less, and removing things that were no longer serving me. I share these lifestyle factors with you in hopes that you'll reflect on your own daily habits and find ways to optimize your health!

Below you'll find the list of lifestyle factors that influence the thyroid. Think of this list as an ongoing check-in! I find that we can always use a bit of fine tuning. Healing never stops and will always be evolving.

5 Important Lifestyle Factors

- Sleep
- Stress
- Endocrine Disruptors
- Diet
- Medications

Lifestyle Factors
That Influence the Thyroid

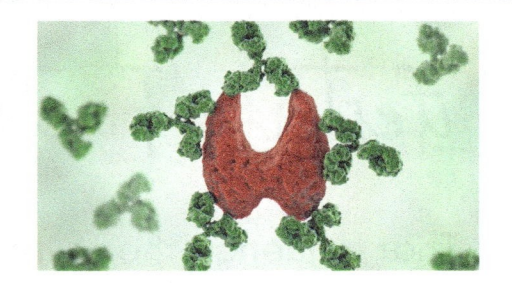

This list on the previous page may seem simple, but it's far from it! The lifestyle component to living with a healthy thyroid has been the hardest part for me due to my anxiety, trauma history, and day to day stress.

That's why I'm constantly searching for more ways to help me de-stress!!

I'm always searching for ways to laugh, fill up my love cup, do things that bring me joy, and to be my authentic true self (setting boundaries, not comparing myself to others and not trying to be someone I'm not!) I'm a girl who loves to hike, garden, to pull weeds, to do arts and crafts, to find free things on Facebook or cheap at garage sales. That's my way of living my happiest life.

What's your way?

I challenge you to write down things that make you feel good and then find ways to make them happen as often as you can! I call this your list of non-negotiables! Use the notes section in the back of the book to write down things that bring you joy.

Lifestyle Factors

That Influence the Thyroid

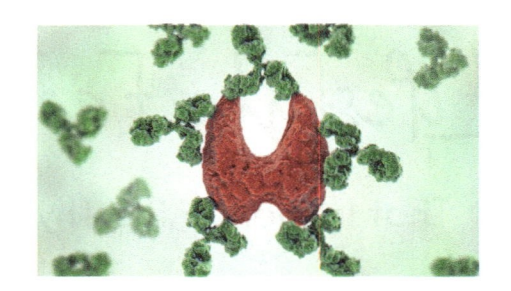

I challenge you to take a moment to reflect on your day. Do you you take time for yourself? Do you plan your meals or snacks so you know what you're eating? Do you stock your pantry and fridge with helpful foods? In chapter twelve, you'll find a blank day for you to fill in. I highly recommend utilizing this tool!

This is just one way to start improving your quality of life while also decreasing negative factors that may influence a thyroid. Let's start with medications.

The list of medications is to encourage you to open a conversation with your doctor, not to discourage you from taking your prescribed meds. Please take your prescribed meds but please be aware of the potential interactions.

Medications that may affect thyroid hormones negatively:

TSH suppression	Inhibition of T4/T3 secretion*	Thyroiditis	TSH elevation	Displacement from thyroxine binding globulin (laboratory artifact)
Glucocorticoids	Lithium	Interferon	Metyrapone	Furosemide
Dopamine agonists	Iodide	Interleukin-2		Phenytoin
Somatostatin analogs	Amiodarone	Amiodarone		Probenecid
Rexinoids	Aminoglutethimide	Sunitinib**		Heparin
Carbemazepine/Oxcarbemazepine				Nonsteroidal anti-inflammatory medications
Metformin				

Thyroid Medication Interactions referenced from
https://www.ncbi.nlm.nih.gov/pmc/articles/PMC2784889/

Lifestyle Factors
That Influence the Thyroid

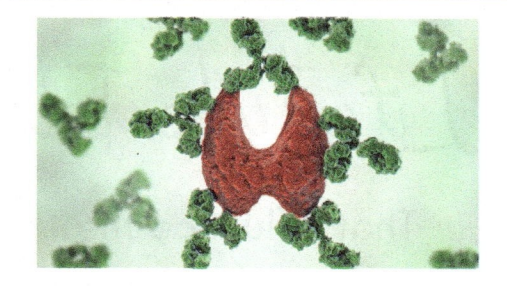

Endocrine Disruptors

There are harmful chemicals that can disrupt hormones. These harmful chemicals can be found in common household items, are preservatives in the foods we eat, and/or are pest deterrents on the produce we eat.

These harmful chemicals are known as endocrine disruptors, endocrine disrupting compounds, or thyroid disrupting chemicals. In my opinion, having three different names for this classification of chemicals/compounds is a direct reflection on the lack of research in the science community. There's new research showing that these compounds are even worse than we first thought.

Endocrine disruptors are man-made chemicals that can disrupt the synthesis, circulating levels, and peripheral action of hormones (8). This means that when you are affected by these chemicals your actual hormones (whether they're made from your own body or in the form of a medication) don't get to their final destination to be used properly. The making of new hormones in your body can also be disrupted.

Lifestyle Factors
That Influence the Thyroid

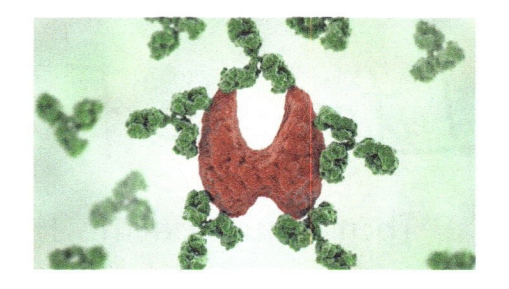

Endocrine Disruptors

Thyroid tissue is very sensitive to endocrine disrupting compounds; it is important to note that iodine deficiency may have the greatest impact on endocrine disruptors influencing thyroid hormones (9). Meaning that if you are not eating enough foods with iodine, then these endocrine disruptors REALLY have a big impact on thyroid hormones.

I can't stress enough that eating a variety of foods is the way to go! Iodine containing foods like seaweed, fish and other seafood, iodized salt, and dairy contains iodine, but I do encourage limiting dairy intake.

However, remember if you have hyperthyroidism you want to limit iodine containing foods. Which means you'll really have to be extra cautious with endocrine disruptors.

I started my journey by removing things like scented wall plugins, changing from scented candles to essential oils, making my own laundry detergent and using wool balls instead of dryer sheets, and changed my self care items over slowly as old ones ran out with better options.

Lifestyle Factors
That Influence the Thyroid

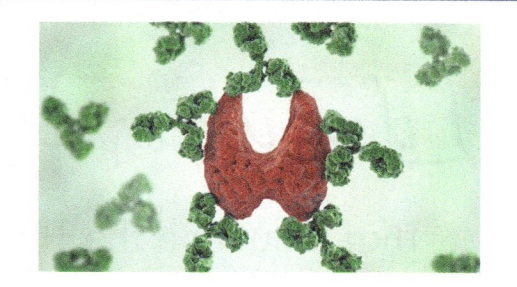

Endocrine Disruptors

I changed my deodorant (I found in the beginning I had to start using a peroxide based face wash or isopropyl alcohol on my arm pits every morning and night to help with smell control, haha), I slowly started changing out my plastic storage containers for glass, and stopped wearing nail polish after my mom got a rare skin cancer under her thumbnail. I replaced my perfume with a mixture of different essential oils, used vinegar to kill weeds in the yard, etc... the list goes on.

One of my favorite sayings is, "I'm doing the best I can with what I have."

Remind yourself of this as you start changing over your products to better choices. You don't have to be perfect or do a complete overhaul. As you're able, start making small changes.

On the next page you'll learn some of the common endocrine disruptors I come up against. And I'll share what I do to minimize my exposure without overwhelming myself by trying to know what ALL these chemicals are. These are only a few and they are listed to encourage you to do your own, now informed, research, so you can make smart choices for you and your family.

Lifestyle Factors
That Influence the Thyroid

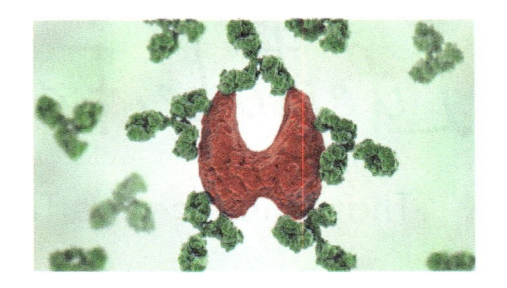

Endocrine disruptors are lurking around the corner at every supermarket, making it difficult to choose products that are a good choice.

I often clean my kitchen with vinegar, water, soap and a few drops of oregano oil. Oregano Oil has been shown to protect against biofilm development (the congregating and coming together of bacteria to make a film) and it also impairs the bacteria's cell membrane (making it useless) (10).

Common Kitchen Endocrine Disruptors
Common endocrine disruptors include, but are not limited to:

- Bisphenols are found in plastics, a common one is BPA or Bisphenol A, however there are many other bisphenols that can cause harm.
    - Dietitian Tips: Always microwave in microwave safe glass and never heat up plastic as this may leach bisphenols into the food.

I have a Products I Trust Page on my website to see what brands I personally use. Visit www.nutritionsmylife.com/products-i-trust or visit www.ewg.org to see if the products you use are a good choice. The EWG is the Environmental Working Group, they research chemicals and brands to provide the public the opportunity to make smart choices.

Lifestyle Factors

That Influence the Thyroid

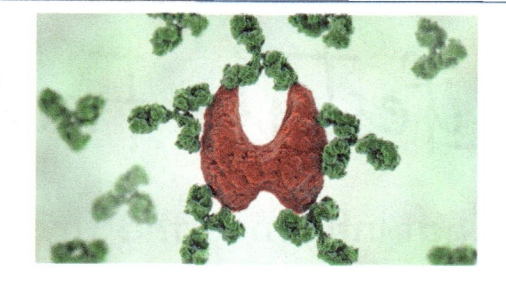

Kitchen Endocrine Disruptors

Common endocrine disruptors include, but are not limited to:

- Phthalates are plasticizer chemicals found in "fragrance," PVC plastic, toys, and plastic wrap.
    - Dietitian Tip: Avoid wrapping hot food in plastic wrap and be aware of the scented soap you use to wash the dishes or in the dishwasher.
    - Drinking water is a common source of exposure for phthalates. Reverse osmosis is helpful.
        - We store our water in a three gallon jug. See my website, wwww.nutritionsmylife.com/products-i-trust page so you can see the container & water system I use (I fill it up at those blue water stations in front of the grocery or convenience stores for just $0.35 a gallon!)
    - Phthalates are also on non-stick pans (try cast iron skillets), in microwavable popcorn, etc.
- Perchlorate, a component of rocket fuel, is an endocrine disruptor that interferes with the thyroid gland and is found in drinking waters and dairy products.

Visit www.nutritionsmylife.com/products-i-trust or visit www.ewg.org to see if the products you use are a good choice.

Lifestyle Factors
That Influence the Thyroid

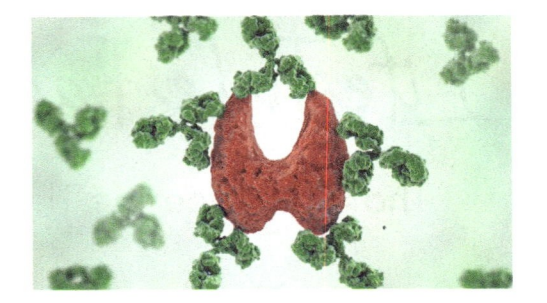

Dermal or skin absorption is the transport of a chemical from the outer surface of the skin both into the skin and into the body (11).

Self-Care Endocrine Disruptors
Common endocrine disruptors include, but are not limited to:

- Parabens are associated with endocrine activity, carcinogens, infertility, spermatogenesis, and psychological and ecological disruptions.
    - When looking for parabens on ingredient labels, look for methylparaben, propylparaben, isoparaben, or butylparaben to avoid.
- Phthalates may be listed as "fragrance" on a variety of products, which is why I read ingredients and avoid all items where fragrances are found. Phthalates are a group of chemicals that will have the word "phthalate" in them. They can be found in nail polish, hair sprays, aftershave lotions, soaps, shampoos, perfumes, and other toiletry items.
- PFAS are warned by the CDC to be harmful to thyroid function (12).

Visit www.nutritionsmylife.com/products-i-trust or visit the www.EWG.org to see if the products you use are a good choice.

Lifestyle Factors

That Influence the Thyroid

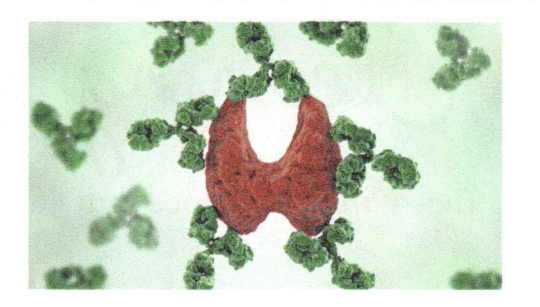

Cleaning the house is important so I try to make as much of my cleaning supplies as I can from scratch. With other cleaning supplies I make sure to avoid the ingredients below.

Cleaning Supplies Endocrine Disruptors

Common endocrine disruptors include, but are not limited to:

- Cyclosiloxanes (e.g. hexamethylcyclotrisiloxane, dodecamethylcyclohexylsiloxane)
- Glycol Ethers (e.g. 2-butoxyethanol, 2,2-methoxyethoxyethanol)
- Phthalates (e.g. DEHP, DEP, DBP)
- Parabens (e.g. methyl paraben, propyl paraben)
- Alkylphenols (e.g. nonylphenols, octylphenols)

Visit www.nutritionsmylife.com/products-i-trust or visit the www.EWG.org website to see if the products you use are a good choice.

Cleaning Supply Recipes

These are the recipes that I use and have not been tested for it's efficacy !

Laundry Detergent

- 3 Gallon Jar to hold it (I currently use a glass jar however I used to use a cleaned out protein powder container.)
- Oxi Clean
- 4lb Box of Baking Soda
- 4lb Box of Washing Soda
- 1lb of Epsom Salt

All Purpose Cleaner

- Empty Spray Bottle
- Fill half-way with water
- Next fill half that amount with distilled white vinegar
- Add a few pumps of soap
- 10 drops of oregano oil

Combine all ingredients in spray bottle and shake well before use.

Chapter Five

Thyroid Challenges

Cortisol & the Thyroid

Elevated cortisol can result in a decrease in thyroid hormones.

Cortisol is one of the steroid hormones and it is made in the adrenal glands. Most cells within the body have cortisol receptors. Cortisol can help control blood sugar levels, regulate metabolism, help reduce inflammation, and assist with memory formulation. It has a controlling effect on salt and water balance, and it helps control blood pressure (13). **Cortisol is helpful for our bodies in the proper amount.**

However, when cortisol levels increase, as they do in high endurance or high intensity workouts where you hit your exhaustion point, this can result in a disruption in thyroid hormones. This is why using yoga, Pilates, a walk, an easy hike, or a leisurely bike ride can be more beneficial for thyroid health than heavy lifting.

This may be conflicting information for a lot of you that want to lose weight. You know that the more muscle mass you have the more energy you're going to expend, meaning a better chance at losing weight. However, heavy weightlifting can only occur once the body is out of the fight or flight response and the thyroid health is stable in an optimal range.

Cliff notes: woosa now / beast mode later

Cortisol & The Thyroid

Choose Low Intensity Workouts

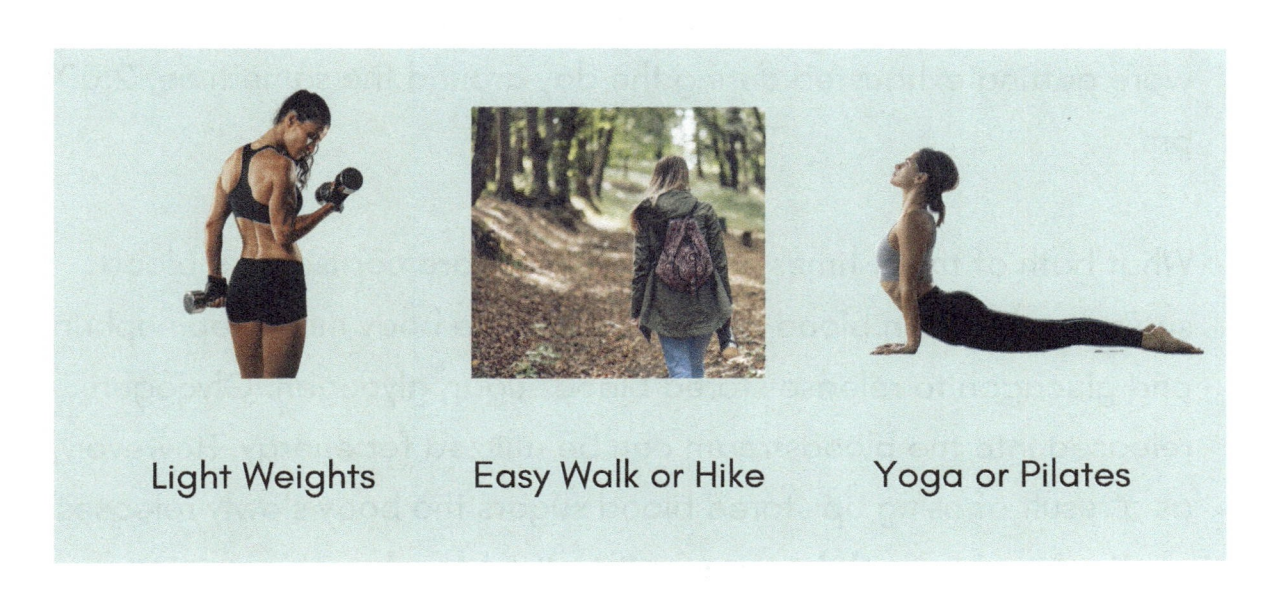

| Light Weights | Easy Walk or Hike | Yoga or Pilates |

Know Your Limits

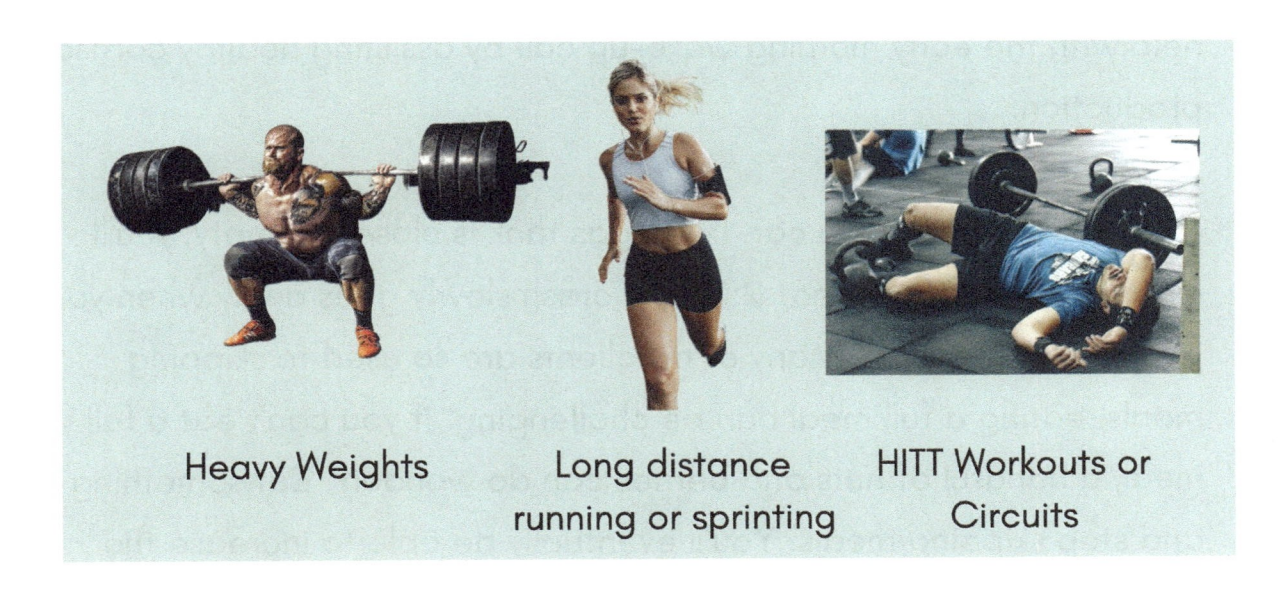

| Heavy Weights | Long distance running or sprinting | HITT Workouts or Circuits |

Healthy Thyroid Guide

Cortisol & The Thyroid

I noticed that many of my clients with hypothyroidism were waking up in the middle of the night around the same time, 2:00-3:00 am, and were getting exhausted during the day around the same time, 2:00 pm.

What both of these times have in common are cortisol and blood sugar levels. When blood sugars are low the body makes epinephrine and glucagon to release stored blood sugar, glycogen. Glycogen released into the bloodstream can be utilized for energy. However, as a result of using up stored blood sugars the body slowly releases **cortisol and growth hormones into the blood.**

Feeding the body enough throughout the day can help stabilize blood sugars and help prevent the 2:00 pm energy crash. It can also help with the early morning wake-up call by assisting healthy cortisol production.

Think of your body as a car. If the gas tank is close to empty, you'll eventually fizzle out. That 2:00 pm crash slowly goes away when you put "fuel in the car!!" Many of my clients are so used to skipping meals, eating a full meal can be challenging. If you can't eat a full meal, a handful of nuts and berries can do wonders. Eat something and stop skipping meals. You'll eventually be able to increase the volume you eat.

Cortisol & The Thyroid

There are many other reasons people have elevated cortisol levels. Some examples include a stressful job, a stressful home environment, a loss of a loved one, a high intensity workout etc.

Getting sunlight in your eyes first thing in the morning to reset your circadian rhythm. This will continue to have the trickle affect of helping you sleep better at night, therefore allowing your body to repair itself. Practicing stress reducing techniques throughout the day is also necessary to allow for healing and repair to happen.

I like to think of this as re-calibration. We're just resetting the body back to factory reset or better known as homeostasis.

Don't underestimate the impact stress has on the body or how powerful stress reducing tools can be, especially the more consistent you are!

Estrogen & The Thyroid

Elevated estrogen can result in a decrease in thyroid hormones.

Estrogen is the other hormone that can have an influence on thyroid hormones. Estrogen increases the thyroxine binding globulin, TBG. TBG binds the thyroid hormones in the blood, therefore an increase in TBG results in a decrease in thyroid hormones in the blood. That means your body doesn't receive the amount it needs (14).

This is why thyroid diseases are more prevalent in women.

In my practice, I see elevated estrogen in women who have poor gut health and also women with PCOS (polycystic ovarian syndrome). Estrogen gets out of our body via the urine and stool (poop). However, sometimes there may be tools lacking to help rid the body of estrogen and then you get a re-uptake of estrogen.

The way to ensure proper estrogen elimination is by eating a diet rich in soluble fiber. Soluble fiber binds to the bile (where estrogen is waiting to be removed in the stool when the time comes) and once the bile is bound to the soluble fiber, it will be eliminated the next time you poop. See the next page for soluble fiber tips.

Knowing your estrogen levels is important, ask your doctor.

Estrogen & The Thyroid

I eat a sweet potato approximately three times a week for breakfast, eat oatmeal for breakfast the other days I'm not eating my sweet potato taco, have a half an avocado almost daily and incorporate broccoli into my dinners each week. All these are great sources of soluble fiber.

Broccoli contains extra estrogen benefits by supporting it's metabolic pathways. A study found that a component in broccoli can reduce cancer risks, specifically estrogen-dominant breast cancer (15). Broccoli sprouts are even more potent than broccoli alone!

Soluble fiber is needed to bind to bile in your intestine. Removal of bile may help lower estrogen and even cholesterol. Below are a few examples of soluble fiber sources to incorporate into your day.

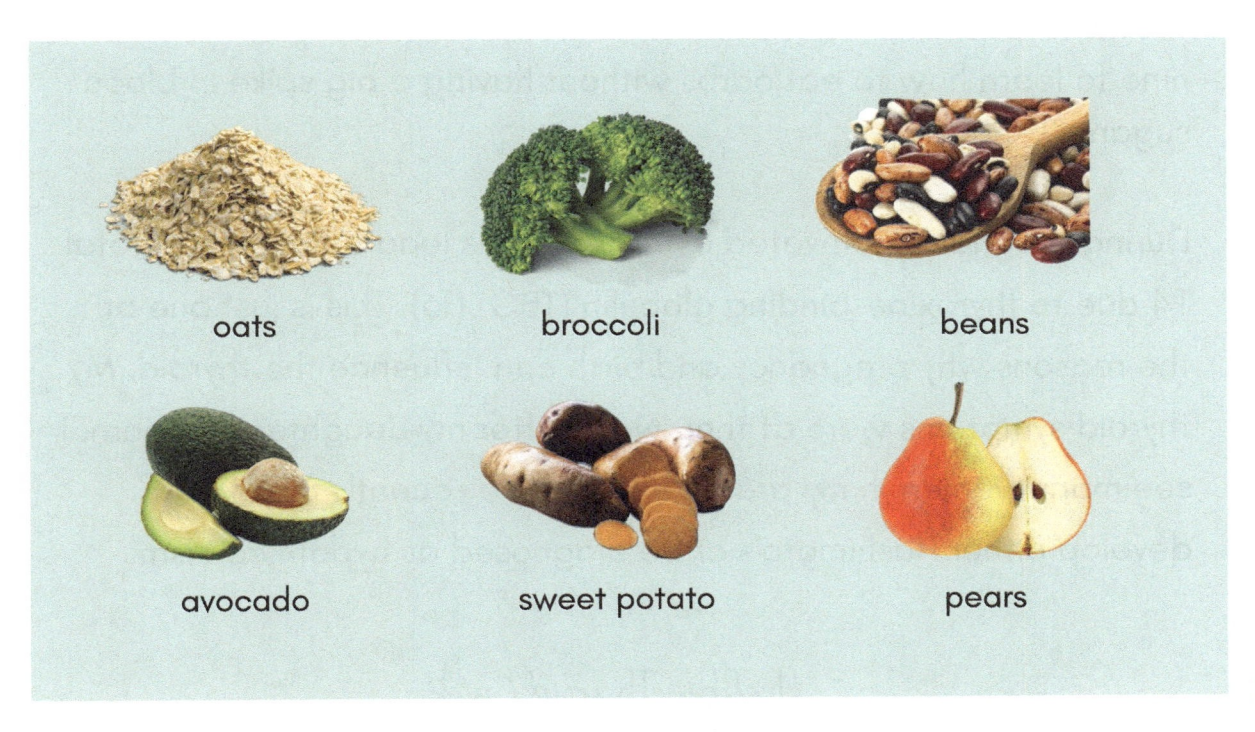

oats   broccoli   beans

avocado   sweet potato   pears

Thyroid & Menstrual Cycles

Did you know there's a correlation between thyroid hormones and reproductive hormones?

Women are more likely to develop thyroid disease than men, and thyroid issues are most common during periods when hormones are changing. That means times like menopause, puberty, and pregnancy. This helps demonstrate the relationship between estrogen and thyroid health (16).

Both hypothyroid and hyperthyroid women have an increase in menstrual disturbances compared with women with normal thyroid levels (16). I see many women that also have polycystic ovarian syndrome (PCOS) develop thyroid disorders due to the elevated estrogen. Note that many people will be placed on the medication, Metformin, for blood sugar control with PCOS. Metformin has been shown to decrease TSH. See the carbohydrate section in chapter nine to learn how to eat carbs without having a big spike in blood sugars.

During pregnancy, elevated estrogen levels lead to increased total T4 due to thyroxine-binding globulin (TBG) (16). This is just one of the reasons why pregnancy and birth can influence the thyroid. My thyroid symptoms were at their worst after my daughter was born. I see many women in my practice that have recently given birth develop either Hashimoto's or be diagnosed as hypothyroidism.

Thyroid & Menstrual Cycles

The thyroid has a strong influence on your menstrual cycle.

The impact of hypothyroidism on the menstrual cycle has been identified since the 1950s and leads to changes in cycle length and blood flow (17).

I remember years ago when my little half a thyroid was still needing Synthroid I ended up having my period three times in the month of November. It was horrible! I didn't know what to do, so I made an appointment with my gynecologist. He told me if I wanted my period regulated, I need to go on birth control.

I luckily said no and he told me to come back when I couldn't handle it anymore...

I then made an appointment with my endocrinologist who told me that my period is regulated by my thyroid. However, he then preceded to tell me that I ought to go on birth control like my gynecologist said because my labs were normal.

(Can I scream through this page?!! He didn't check ALL my labs nor my reproductive hormones)

Now that you know the thyroid has a role in your menstrual cycle, be your own advocate and ask for more labs... ASK WHY did this happen, not just HOW to fix it (even though the fix would have been just a band aide).

Thyroid & Menstrual Cycles

In my opinion, birth control has it's time and place but it get's over prescribed. It has been shown that oral contraceptives depletes folic acid, vitamins B2, B6, B12, vitamin C and E and the minerals magnesium, selenium, and zinc (18). Remember in chapter one how we discussed the importance of selenium and zinc in the role of thyroid hormones?

Magnesium has over 300 roles in the body and if low, causes increase in anxiety, stress, headaches or migraines, constipation, muscle spasms, and weakness to name a few.

B vitamins play a role in our energy and also in our nervous system. B vitamins also play a role in helping the body rid itself of histamine (hello allergies). They also play a role in making red blood cells. Low red blood cells means anemia and anemia negatively affects the thyroid.

When oral contraceptives are given out like candy versus finding the root cause, you can see how "fixing" one problem can lead to many other issues. I'm a big fan of finding the root cause, figuring out what's going on, and giving the body the tools to repair itself.

Yes, oral contraceptives are helpful for many. Yes, oral contraceptives can help symptoms. Yes, they have their time and place but I see the over prescribing of medication as a dangerous thing.

Now, this is not me saying stop your meds but educate yourself and to empower yourself to ASK more questions!

Thyroid & Menopause

Menopause results in a drop in estrogen.

Which can make you feel like your thyroid symptoms are so much worse!!

Some women who go through menopause struggle with their energy, libido, and weight loss. Tack on a thyroid disorder and this combination takes a toll on their bodies. Women may also have a difficult time with their emotions in the sense of being "short tempered" during this time.

I see this so often in my practice and there's a few things we can do to help support the thyroid and menopause symptoms. It comes from the foods we choose to feed our bodies every day and it comes through healthy habits that we work to consistently be our best at, while also giving ourselves grace when we aren't able to accomplish the goals you set out to do.

Foods that support hormone health are the healthy fats. These are essential fatty acids like those found in nuts, seeds, avocado, olives, olive oil, grass-fed beef, fatty fish, fish oil, and the best one for reproductive health is in a supplement called evening primrose oil.

Evening primrose oil is extremely high in two types of fats called, linoleic acid (LA) and y-linolenic acid (GLA). These fats are the precursors towards the anti-inflammatory pathway (19). Evening primrose oil also contains polyphenols, which are a component of plants and act similarly to antioxidants. They help in defense against ultraviolet radiation or aggression by pathogens (20). **It's so cool that eating plants or supplements derived from plants supports our bodies because of the plant's built in self-defense mechanisms!**

Thyroid & Menopause
Menopause results in a drop in estrogen.

Estrogens influence the immune and inflammatory processes. Which, lucky us, correlates to why women are more susceptible to infection, sepsis, and higher rate of autoimmune diseases than men. Women also have a higher rate of different chronic inflammatory disease during the menstrual cycle, pregnancy, and menopause (21).

What this means that estrogen helps keep the inflammation at bay. When the estrogen is low, you feel more aches and pains.

The thyroid does not like inflammation. In fact I want you to always be thinking, "Am I eating enough anti-inflammatory fats throughout the day?" and also, "Do I have enough color in my meals?" These two questions can help ensure you're eating enough essential fatty acids and antioxidants, polyphenols and flavonoids to help with inflammation reduction. See how the thyroid is connected to almost every part of our bodies!!??

Estrogen levels impact inflammation which impacts the thyroid.

One thing that I like to do is provide low estrogen with supportive foods like soy. Even though they have estrogen like properties, they can also block the more potent estrogen from attaching to the receptor, helping to reduce estrogen levels if elevated. Chapter eight discusses soy in more depth.

Thyroid & Menopause

The type of soy does matter. I only buy organic tofu or edamame when I'm at the grocery store; this is due to glyphosate. Glyphosate is the most widely used herbicide worldwide. A meta analysis study linked exposures to glyphosate-based herbicides and increased risk for non-Hodgkin's lymphoma (22). I've already had 2 cancer scares; I don't want another and that's my reason for going organic.

Soy patties, protein powders and soy chicken nuggets need to be left off the menu. I tend to opt out of fake chicken and choose a meal or recipe with beans or tofu if going for a meatless option. This means have fun experimenting with different tofu recipes!! Edamame also makes for an easy snack. I shared a tofu recipe in this guide just so you have some guidance on how to make healthy taste good.

I recommend choosing legumes (beans, peas, or lentils) most of the time when searching for meatless options.

Seed Cycling

In addition to incorporating soy to support the low estrogen that typically is associated with menopause, an additional option is seed cycling. In seed cycling you use seeds to mimic the rise and fall of women's hormones through the month.

Sounds really cool right? Eat some seeds and balance your hormones! This isn't just for menopausal women, but ALL women, unless otherwise specified by doctor, may find benefits in seed cycling for various reasons.

An estrogen boost is what helps control the growth of the uterine lining during the first part of the cycle, the follicular phase. If a woman's egg is not fertilized, estrogen levels decrease sharply and menstruation begins. Milled flaxseed and pumpkin seeds should be eaten during this phase.

During the luteal phase of the menstrual cycle (the day you ovulate to the day you start your period) has an increase in progesterone and drop in estrogen. Sesame and sunflower seeds may be beneficial during this part of the cycle.

Since menopausal women don't have their periods, you can start this at any time. See next page for the visual on how to do this and note, most of my clients start to notice a difference around month two to three. Consistency is key!

Seed Cycling

Day 1-13
Estrogen Boost

(menstrual + follicular phase. aka day 1 of your period)

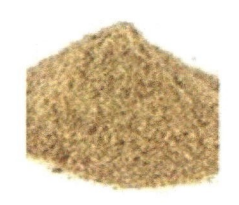

1 Tbsp a day of Milled/ground Flax seed

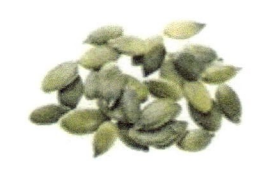

1 Tbsp a day of Pumpkin Seeds

Day 14-28
Progresterone Boost

(Ovulation + Luteal Phase)

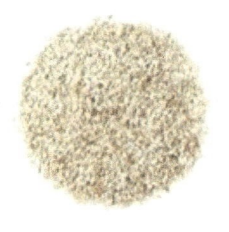

1 Tbsp a day of Sesame Seeds

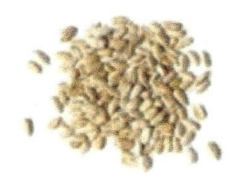

1 Tbsp a day of Sunflower Seeds

Thyroid and Men

Thyroid disorders are more prevalent in women than in men. In fact one in eight women will have a thyroid disorder in their lifetime. **Women are five to eight times more likely than men to have thyroid problems.**

However, thyroid disorders DO happen in men and what you're learning from this Healthy Thyroid Guide applies to you if you're male! The only thing I'd hold off on is the seed cycling discussed earlier in this chapter.

Testosterone is known as the "male hormone" and is important for normal development and function of male reproductive organs. Free testosterone concentrations are reduced in men with primary **hypothyroidism** and thyroid hormone replacement normalizes free testosterone concentrations (23). If a young male has hypothyroidism, they may not develop their gonads properly. Therefore it is crucial to seek medical attention for boys with thyroid issues.

Men with **hyperthyroidism** tend to have elevated concentrations of testosterone and sex hormone binding globulin, which can lead to many other health problems (acne, mood swings, irritability, headaches, insomnia, increase risk of heart attack, increase risk of blood clots etc.)

Thyroid and Transgender

With the rise in people transitioning from male to female or female to male in the LGBTQ community, I wanted to include research for this population. However, there is very little research that I could find and I have no experience with this population, to be completely transparent.

Estrogen and androgen therapy has been shown to decrease the conversion of T4 to T3 due to rising estrogen from medication causing an increase in TBG hormones, as we previously discussed in this chapter can have a decrease in available T4. However, this was found to only occur with oral estrogen replacement and not transdermal, through the skin (23).

Testosterone replacement therapy has been shown to decrease TBG and cause an increase in the T4 to T3 conversion (24).

Male transitioning to female may be at higher risk for thyroid dysfunction than females transitioning to male.

If I had a client who is undergoing their transition or had transitioned, I'd want to know their thyroid labs and their pituitary status. The pituitary gland influences nearly every part of the body and the hormones it produces help regulate important functions like growth, reproductive health, and blood pressure even.

Working closely with an endocrinologist is important and a dietitian who specializes in endocrinology may be beneficial as well.

Chapter Six

Thyroid Challenges Part Two
- Thyroid Weight Loss
- Sleep
- Stress
- Hair Loss

Thyroid Weight Loss

What I have to say about thyroid weight loss may go against what you see on social media. Calorie restriction is not going to work. Reducing your calories drastically can result in changes in your thyroid function.

Division of Endocrinology and Metabolism, Department of Internal Medicine, University of Michigan Medical School presented these results:

> Treatment of obesity with hypocaloric diets causes changes in thyroid function that resemble sick euthyroid syndrome. Changes consist of a decrease in total T4 and total and free T3 with a corresponding increase in reverse T3 (25).

My favorite analogy to help you understand why restricting calories or skipping meals (which technically is restricting calories) is harmful is **"the hibernating bear."** Hear me out... When a bear hibernates, its metabolism has to slow down to conserve energy. It doesn't have energy coming in because it's sleeping. The body is amazing and conserves energy by slowing down it's basal metabolic rate or BMR. BMR is the amount of energy expended at rest.

This survival mechanism is the same thing that happens for many people, especially those with a thyroid disorder. Cutting calories will not work as this will further slow down the BMR. (i.e. someone with a low BMR of 1000 calories will gain weight if eating 1200 calories a day.. which 1200 calories is the amount for a toddler).

What about working out to lose weight!? There was a study that demonstrated how working out until exhaustion caused a negative effect on the thyroid for up to 24hrs post workout (26). Avoiding high intensity workouts while you're repairing your thyroid and BMR can be beneficial in the long run. Choose yoga, Pilates, and walking. Once you're not in a state of stress and have given your body enough time to reset your BMR, then and only then should you include heavy weight lifting or high intensity workouts.

Thyroid Weight Loss

Everything that is in this guide is applicable for thyroid weight loss. There will be a time eventually (and I stress EVENTUALLY) where you'll be able to cut back a few carbohydrates for weight loss (I said a few) and will eventually be able to begin to lift heavier weights. But it is not going to happen until all the following have been addressed...consistently. *An increase in appetite typically means less inflammation and improved metabolism*!

Thyroid Weight Loss Non-Negotiables

- Foundation anti-inflammatory diet
- Plate method used at every meal & portion sizes are followed
- Nutrient demands met for your specific health conditions (thyroid nutrients are listed in chapter nine)
- Stress reduction (the body won't release weight when stress is present)
- Sleep (deep sleep achieved most nights with minimum of 7-8 hours slept each night is crucial for weight loss)
- Exercise is appropriate for the phase you're in
    - Early in your repair / healing journey: light exercises like walking, stretching, yoga, and Pilates
    - Months of consistency, labs improved, feeling well: start incorporating heavier weightlifting and/or high intensity workouts.

Thyroid Weight Loss

Losing weight with a thyroid disorder means you might gain weight before you lose weight.

The BMR must be reset and the only way to do that is to consistently feed your body nutritious meals. In order to feed yourself properly, with the appropriate nutrients, you may increase your current caloric intake.

Weight gain may be a temporary side effect of resetting your BMR.
What I have found from the people I work with that have a thyroid disorder is that it takes months for weight loss to occur, but let me tell you what you need to do so it will happen. *Stop weighing yourself so much and get the measuring tape out or take monthly pictures.* **Keep focused on how you're feeling, what you are feeding your body, reducing stress, and being consistent.** Over time you'll slowly increase your BMR, so you'll burn more calories at rest and will help with your weight loss goals.

Case Study: I had a client try for months to lose weight . She has a thyroid disorder, has stress/anxiety and digestive issues. She wasn't seeing the scale budge but she did notice more energy, better sleep, less joint pain. She worked at her health for three solid months. Finally was able to start working out and lost 2.5cm from her waist, without the scale budging! She eventually lost the weight she wanted but for months nothing happened on the scale but her body was changing. If she would have just focused on the scale and nothing else, she would have missed out on her progress and maybe even given up.

> If you have been consistent with all these tools for a month or two and want to start the weight loss process, I'd suggest a slight reduction in carbohydrates at dinner time only. I'm not saying carb free but instead of 1/2 cup of carbohydrates, it's now 1/4 cup carbohydrates. Breakfast and lunch + snacks will remain appropriate serving sizes.

Thyroid Weight Loss

If you're not losing weight and you feel like you're doing everything listed on the previous page then...

Let's pinpoint what may be happening here:

____ Can you honestly say your stress is under control?
Stress could be from not sleeping, stress could be from your job, stress could be chemical, emotional, or physical. Stress could be anxiety or stress could be overwhelmed. I see stress as a major inhibiting factor for many people. If stress is improved, consistent nutrient demands have been met and you actually feel hungrier and have more energy, *then try decreasing dinner's carbohydrate from 1/2 cup to 1/4 cup.*

____ How long have you been consistent with all of these thyroid supporting tools?

For some people, a month is long enough to start seeing weight loss and for others it take three months or longer, until it happens. Keep in mind how much repair the body needs to do! *Did you give it enough time to reset and repair?* More than likely, you're doing many things that are right but you just have to be patient with the process. Keep focusing on how you're feeling! If you have more energy, are sleeping better, have less achy joints, and improved digestion... then you're on the right road! Keep the consistency going, time will be your best friend!! If you're not feeling much better, it may be time to set up a one on one session with a dietitian so they can see what else could be going on.

Thyroid and Sleep

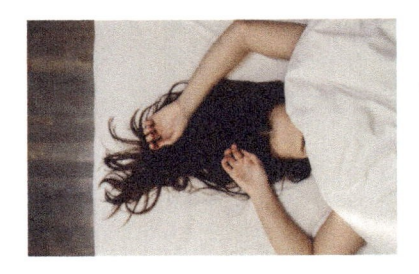

I'm a big advocate for sleep!

It used to be something that eluded me for many years and I occasionally still have problems at night. We're creatures of habits and this is exactly how our sleep works with the circadian rhythm.

Circadian rhythms are physical, mental, and behavioral changes that follow a 24-hour cycle (27). These natural processes respond primarily to light and dark. One example of a light-related circadian rhythm is sleeping at night and being awake during the day.

Circadian rhythms can influence important functions in our bodies in addition to sleep, such as:

hormone release,
eating habits and digestion,
body temperature

Thyroid and Sleep

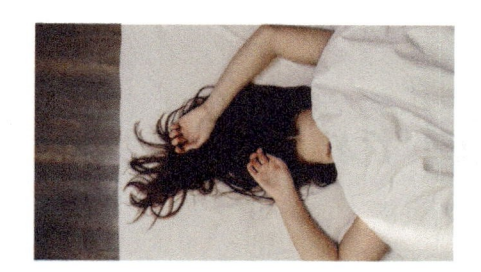

However, what happens to many people is that you wake up, get ready for work/school/the day, and then blaze through your day. But you end up feeling burnt out around 2-4 pm. What happened in the morning? Answer is, there was no sunlight to set your circadian rhythm. This is why it's so important to take some time outside every morning, or if that's not doable based on your work schedule or location, a sunlamp in your bathroom may be a helpful investment.

What also tends to happen when we go outside? Sunglasses immediately go on when you step outside. I attended a brain health conference where the speaker shared a great stress hack that can be done at the same time you're doing your morning circadian rhythm set. Take off your sunglasses for 20 minutes a day to receive sunlight directly into your eyes for stress and anxiety reduction. If depression is present spend an extra 10 minutes a day for a total of 30 minutes of sunlight. I'm not saying look at the sun but step out into the sun's warmth.

Mental health is a big factor in whether you're going to get a good night's sleep or not. For some people chronic stress can cause them to wake up in the middle of the night around 2-4 am. Some people have a difficult time with falling asleep due anxiety or depression.

Thyroid and Sleep

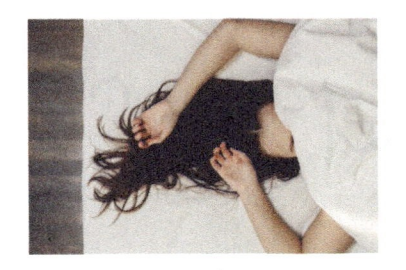

That morning sunlight is crucial for our circadian rhythm but sunlight in general is crucial for our health...and I'm not even talking vitamin D yet!

Exposure to both UVA and UVB radiation may help prevent autoimmune diseases (28). Yes you read that right, sunlight may help prevent autoimmune diseases. This is because these rays, UVA and UVB, removes the actual cell that makes autoimmune diseases.

Sunlight in the form of UVR, increases blood levels of natural opiates called endorphins (28). Endorphins make you feel good which helps you stress less. Stress can definitely be a culprit in keeping someone awake at night. Reducing stress is a great way to help you fall asleep easier.

During my struggles with anxiety, panic attacks, unbalanced hormones, and inflammation it could take me three to four hours to fall asleep. Which meant I'd only sleep four to five hours. I wasn't receiving the repair at night my body desperately needed. I was also waking up early to go to work and not spending the time in the sun like my body needed.

Thyroid and Sleep

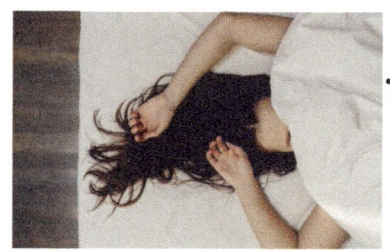

I found that decreasing my caffeine intake was helpful, and the same time I started falling in love with my morning routine. Initially I needed to almost have a ritual-like routine where I'd make my turmeric latte, go into my office, and light the meditation candles. I would sit in my comfy chair and start my meditation music. Then I would get lost in thought, refocus on my breath, then get lost in thought again.

Meditation was difficult at first but it eventually became a practice to help me stress less. I was getting better but still not where I knew I needed to be.

I continued to keep searching for more helpful tools and will never stop.

I noticed that the days where I didn't start a morning routine of some sort were the same days where I struggled with sleep the most. I started noticing this with my clients as well!

My mornings look different now but it still starts outside. Now, I take time to tend to my garden. Start an outdoor morning routine if you're able and make it your own.

Thyroid and Sleep

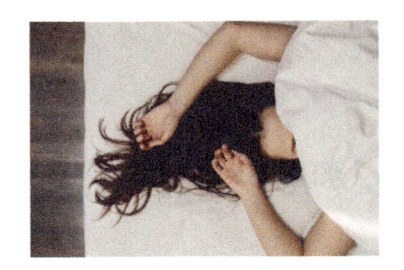

When you're rushed to get out of the door or tending to everyone else's need, there is no calm or time for yourself.

Taking time to be calm and grateful in the morning can help set the tone for the day. This seems like such a simple step but it's missed by so many. I understand there is a lot to do in a day, but you know what? There will always be something left to do, always something to add to the to do list, and always something that doesn't get done off that to do list. We feel we have to have superpowers to do it all but in reality this mentality is a major part of the problem.

I like to say, if you want to do repairs on a car and it's flying down the highway at 100 MPH, you'll crash and burn! This is how I like to envision the body. If we don't take time to slow down that car in the morning, you'll eventually crash and burn at some point during your day.

Take time throughout the day even to cool off that engine. I often take stretching breaks or just breaks to stand outside to take deep belly breathes. This helps regulate the hypothalamus, pituitary, and adrenal axis as well. Which plays a huge role in hormone health and sleep patterns.

Thyroid and Sleep

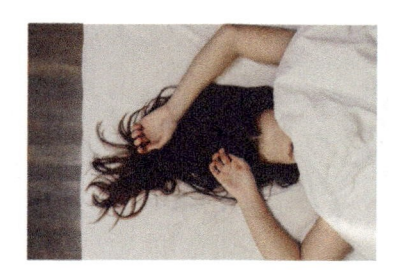

I also see people who don't eat enough throughout the day or don't eat enough at dinner. This causes them to wake up in the middle of the night due to a dip in blood glucose levels (blood sugars). This typically results in a release of cortisol which stimulates the release of glycogen (stored blood sugars). Ever feel like you get jolted awake? You're feeling the cortisol and big spike in blood sugars.

Alcohol, caffeine consumed after noon, and blue light are three common deep sleep disruptors that should be addressed to help improve quality of sleep. I have built in blue light canceling into my prescription glasses. There are many different ones you can get to go over your current glasses, or if you don't wear glasses, they have great options for blue light canceling glasses! With the amount of screen time we're getting daily, we need to eliminate as much as possible and an easy way is by wearing blue light canceling glasses.

It's easy to see why so many people struggle with sleep, when there's so many factors that go into getting a good quality night's sleep!

Let's not negotiate your health anymore! Check out the Sleep Better Non-Negotiables on the next page to help you catch some zzzz's.

Better Sleep Non-Negotiables

- Sunlight every morning

- Stress reduction tools throughout the day

- Eat balanced meals and eat enough throughout the day to help stabilize blood sugar

- Avoid caffeine after noon (deep sleep disruptor)

- Avoid alcohol too close to bedtime (deep sleep disruptor)

- Blue light canceling glasses (deep sleep disruptor)

- Epsom salt baths (magnesium rich to help relax)

- Eat cherries as they naturally contain melatonin

- Journal or write out your todo list for tomorrow

Thyroid and Stress

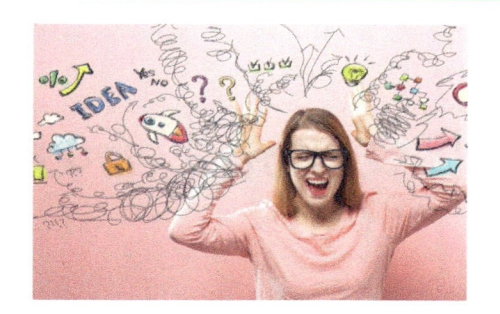

Have you tried working out really hard to lose weight or just become healthier and nothing...no results?! It could be because your body was already in a state of stress and then you added more stress to it. Yes, working out is a stress reliever but if you're not sleeping well, not happy in a job or a relationship, frustrated with yourself over your health, have inflammation or digestive issues, etc... if the body is in the sympathetic nervous system (this is the fight or flight response) repairing, anabolism (building of muscles, build up of metabolism, etc.), increased energy, and achieving weight loss will be difficult. If the body is getting put in to the sympathetic nervous system at a high rate, it may be having a bigger impact on your health than you think.

Elevated cortisol levels such as seen in people that workout until exhaustion have shown a correlation with increased TSH (26). Cortisol is a stress hormone and is helpful in small amounts. The problem lies in too much cortisol or elevations at the wrong time of day.

Inflammation is another big stress to the thyroid and it's one of the "Was it the chicken or the egg first scenario" because stress induces inflammation and inflammation induces stress.

Thyroid and Stress

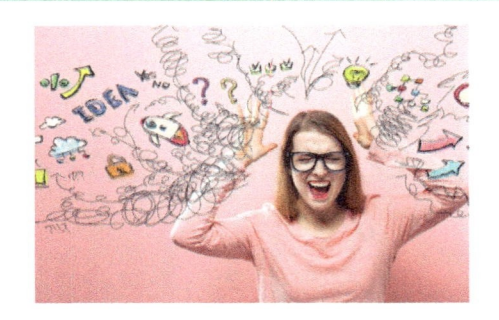

I've seen people with normal C-reactive protein (CRP: Inflammatory protein marker in the blood) and elevated retinol binding protein (RBP: Inflammation protein marker in the blood). No matter if you have current inflammation or not, I still encourage everyone to be on an anti-inflammatory diet. This is because it can help PREVENT inflammation as well.

Yes! We can prevent things from happening inside our body! For example, I can prevent the frequency and severity of my anxiety by following a lot of what's discussed in this book and on the stress less non-negotiable checklist. I'm able to prevent frequency and severity of migraines. **The body wants to repair and work for us, sometimes it just is like a shopping cart at the grocery store... if you don't keep putting some effort into it, it'll veer off and crash into something.**

You must tackle stress and inflammation at the same time!! Just like you have to tackle stress and digestive health at the same time. Anxiety and stress can cause the blood flow to be shunted from the intestines to the muscles. This is why many people who are stressed or anxious also suffer with digestive issues.

Thyroid and Stress

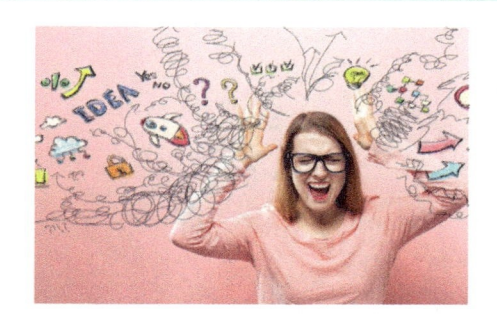

What's one thing you could do every day that brings you joy? I challenge you to seek out joy! Joy means you're living in the moment. Joy means you're not in a current state of stress.

Throughout this Healthy Thyroid Guide, you've read stress reduction a few times. Most people will either say yes to having a lot of stress or no, I don't have stress. The "no, I don't have stress" people tend to have multiple health issues and are the ones who end up having the most stress in my experience. I find this is due to people thinking that having every minute of their day full is normal. Or they use other words like over-stimulated or busy. However, stress is not just having a lot to do.

**There are 3 different types of stress:
Emotional, Physical, and Chemical.**

Emotional Stress can be from depression and anxiety, it can be from a difficult relationship, or even be the loss of a loved one, amongst many other things.

Physical Stress could be childbirth, a car accident, recent surgery (although surgery & childbirth may also have some chemical stress), exercising too much or too intense, a physically demanding job, anorexia, calorie restriction or dieting.

Thyroid and Stress

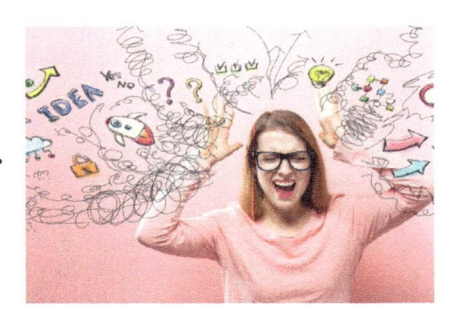

Chemical stress can occur from inhaling perfumes, scented candles, exhaust from a car, harmful cleaning supplies, etc. Chemical stress can occur from exposure to bisphenol containing plastics, the perfumes in lotions, fragrances in body washes, and make-ups even. Chemical stress can occur from caffeine or the processed foods we eat.

Stress can be so many different things and it's not fair to say, "well I only have xyz wrong with me, and they have been through xyz ...." Please don't compare yourself to other people. Stress is stress. It's real to you. It's a big deal to you, so stop ignoring it.

Understanding and labeling stress is one thing but taking action is another. Let's walk through some tips I do personally and recommend to my clients as well.

Say anxiety or depression is your body's constant stressor. Start doing things like eating more magnesium rich foods, taking magnesium glycinate or magnesium threonate, taking fish oil with extra DHA (as most studies recommend 1-2g/day of DHA), eating consistently throughout the day, and incorporating stress reducing habits, like starting your day outside or with some form of sunlight. Sunlight is a great way to reduce stress by helping set the circadian rhythm. Taking time to be outside is really forgotten by many.

Thyroid and Stress

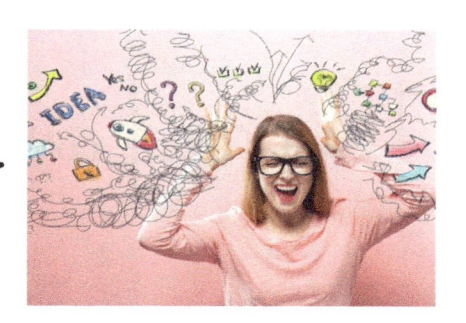

I can't tell you how many people I talk to each week that don't get outside most days. Getting outside isn't just about vitamin D but connecting to the earth and grounding yourself. Nature brings back peace.

Another stress reduction hack is the stress flame!
I like to visualize stress as a flame when I get stressed. I do this because if I don't put out that stress flame, it will soon set me on fire. This prompts me to stop at that moment and do something to de-stress, like a quick dance party, deep breaths, or a walk outside.

The stress flame is an important visualization tool that helps remind you to check in with yourself and to help regulate your emotions.

Stress Case Study #1: I had a client that was seeing me for hypothyroidism and digestive health. She was doing well with her food intake and making sure she was meeting her nutrient demands with food. However, she wasn't able to lose any weight, which was a big goal of hers. Yes, she was seeing an improvement in her digestion, energy and sleep but she wasn't fully there yet with her stress. One session I asked, "What's something you haven't done in a while that you really enjoy?" She said, "Taking pictures! I used to take the most beautiful pictures but haven't picked up my camera in a long time. I just don't have the time for it."

Thyroid and Stress

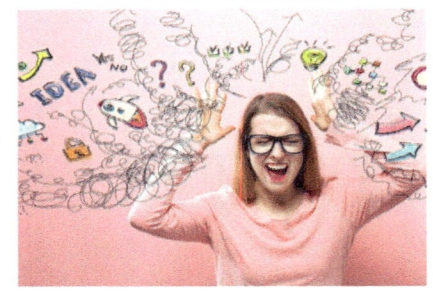

We discussed different times throughout the week where she might be able to find some time and by the next session, she was finding time almost daily because it was so fun for her.

Guess what happened the following session? She told me she lost weight! She had all the tools finally in alignment with her body's needs. The last missing puzzle piece was stress.

Stress Case Study #2: I had a client who had a transformation after she addressed stress. This thyroid warrior had no thyroid and was working diligently to improve her inflammation, support her thyroid with the thyroid supporting foods, and improve her gut health, but was not handling stress very well.

I asked her what she felt like the major stressor in her life was, and she actually said it was her mother. She ended up having a conversation with her mom and started to rebuild their relationship. She dropped two pants sizes after that.

I will say it again and again: Stress is like a gremlin that lives on your shoulder. It has to be addressed.

Thyroid and Stress

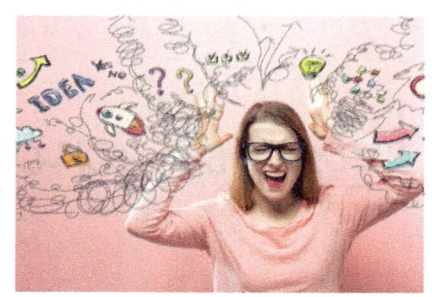

This might be repetitive but stressing less is KEY! My life really started changing for the better when I began searching for ways to learn how to stress less and tackle my anxiety.

I would meditate in the morning with an essential oil diffusing or a drop on my neck to bring me to a happier place. The smell always had cloves in it because cloves reminds me of doing arts and crafts with my mom when I was younger. Then, I'd take that essential oil with me throughout the day by wearing it on lava rock jewelry or directly on my skin.

Meditation makes you feel good. The scent makes me feel good and memory is tied to scent. If you wear the smell that you had on while you meditate, you'll be able to smell your essential oil and be reminded of feeling good.

This trick has helped me when I've gone to the zoo, when I've had an important meeting, or going to a concert... all places where my anxiety usually hits hard. It helps so much!

Thyroid and Anxiety

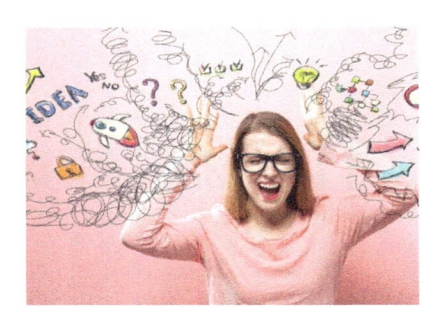

Anxiety is extremely common with thyroid disorders and is extremely stressful to the body and thyroid.

Anxiety can occur due to a few reasons like poor gut health, inflammation, lack of key nutrients (B vitamins, magnesium, and omega 3 fatty acids), and even from the thyroid causing irregular heart beats.

When I was on my thyroid hormone replacement medication, I had many heart palpitations and it freaked me out! I remember having panic attacks and even though I knew they were panic attacks, I still felt like I was having a heart attack. Anxiety also causes an elevated heart rate. My trick for this is to tell yourself you're excited.

When you're excited, heart rate increases and you can even get sweaty palms and butterflies. It takes repetition to really feel like this makes a difference but try telling yourself, "I'm excited, I'm excited!" It helps me, and has helped me since writing this guide for you. I couldn't believe I was actually doing this and almost started spiraling, but then caught myself a few thoughts in.

Thyroid and Stress

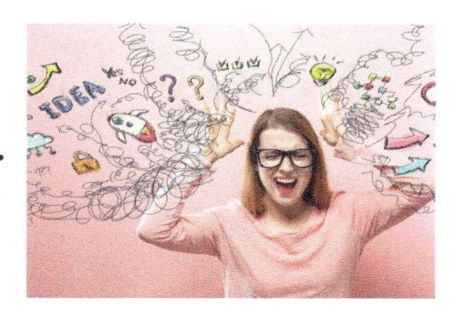

My anxiety talk that goes on in my head is called Bertha. Bertha, to me, is someone nasty. She's an unhappy woman whose sole purpose in life is to make me miserable.

I get to separate myself from Bertha and get to tell her to stop talking, to leave me alone, and even to shut up! I've had a client label her anxiety "that annoying frat boy." Whatever works for you, works! The role of labeling your anxiety is to help separate yourself from the anxiety, so you're able to think clearer.

I had the privilege of quitting a job that made me unhappy and start working for myself, which allows me the time I need to practice stress reduction daily. I'd encourage you to take a look at your day to find time for yourself every day and then also add something big to look forward to. You really are worth spending time on.

When I was starting out, I'd listen to motivational speakers on YouTube and even went to a conference of one of them. Do what feels right at the time to help you learn the tools to stress less.
I see a therapist once a month and if you need to, reach out to one! I can't stress enough how important it is to take care of your stress.

Stress Less Non-Negotiables

-Gratitude
[start while in your bed & then carry gratitude throughout the day, you may need to set reminders on your phone at first]

- Sunlight every morning

- Remove or reduce stressful things
[caffeine, start saying NO sometimes, stop comparing, put the scale away etc]

- Schedule YOU time every day
[20 minutes can go a long way. Grab it when you can]

- Learn how smother the stress flame in the moment
[jumping up and down, dancing, learning how to box breathe etc]

- Eat enough throughout the day
[using the plate method & eating consistently throughout the day will help stabilize blood sugars- this helps reduce inflammation which is key in stress reduction]

- Meet your magnesium demands through foods, supplements, and yes,

- Unscented epsom salt baths [Magnesium rich to help relax]

- Make sleep a priority

- Journal or write out your to-do list for tomorrow
[this is especially helpful right before bed]

Thyroid Hair Loss

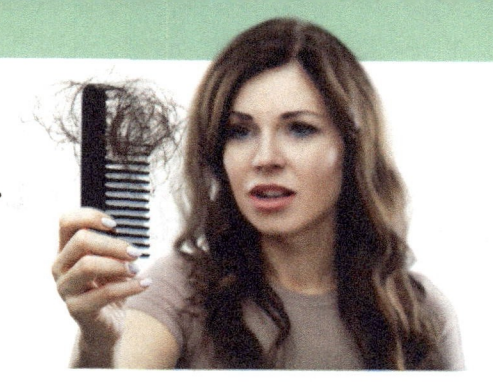

The thyroid controls the hair follicle's stimulation for new growth (aka the hair's metabolism). For most people who have hair loss associated with hypothyroidism, it's due to hair falling out at a normal rate but it being slow to grow in. Your hair's metabolism is too slow to grow back the new hair.

Improve your thyroid's health and your hair will start to grow back at it's normal rate. However, this can take months to happen! If thyroid hair loss is something that you would like to improve, supporting the thyroid of course helps. But you can still support hair health with a few other things not yet discussed in this thyroid guide. This information also applies to nail growth, as well.

Biotin is well known to support nail and hair growth but caution needs to be taken in thyroid warriors when it comes to supplementation, especially if you're getting your labs drawn. Taking biotin may cause hyperthyroid levels without symptoms (29). I do not recommend biotin supplementation in thyroid warriors. Instead, eat foods rich in biotin. Biotin is found in chicken, eggs, carrots, broccoli, spinach, sweet potatoes, bananas, avocado, strawberries, walnuts, and many more. The body loves a variety of food.

Thyroid Hair Loss

Sulphur is an important mineral in our body. Sulphur is necessary in the steps to make keratin hair protein and is a key element in growing hair (30). Sulphur rich foods include onions, garlic, green leafy vegetables, cabbage, broccoli, avocado, nuts, and sweet potatoes.

Healthy fats also play an in important role in hair growth. This is why I encourage all my clients to have a source of healthy fats at every meal and most snacks too. The fats we eat play a role in making hormones and this helps keep hair in the outer skin layer (30). Healthy fat options are avocado, nuts, seeds, olives, olive oils, fatty fish, pasture raised eggs, and grass-fed beef.

Stress reduction is a must but again, we knew that lol. Reducing your stress levels by incorporating more fun, gratitude, and happiness into your life can have a big impact.

Hair growth can happen, but it takes time, just like most health journeys.

Chapter Seven

Thyroid Supporting Nutrients

Thyroid Supporting Nutrients

In this part of the book, you'll start to understand how different foods can support a healthy thyroid.

Make note that when I mention "healthy thyroid" throughout this guide, I'm referring to more than just the thyroid gland. I'm referring to proper synthesis or making of thyroid hormones and communication of the thyroid hormones with the body. Healthy thyroid even applies if you're a halfy like me, or you don't have a thyroid at all, because the thyroid medication you take still needs to communicate and work well inside the body.

This guide is intended to be an educational tool, not medical advice. Please see your doctor and/or registered dietitian before starting a new diet and health regimen.

Thyroid Supporting Nutrients

Selenium

I have a few stories about selenium that always come to mind. The first is about a professor of mine back in college. He studied selenium, wrote his own biochemistry book, and traveled the world helping people purify water with selenium. This mineral always fascinated me because of his passion for it. I could have never imagined back then how big of an impact this mineral would have on my career as dietitian or even on my own personal health.

The other story is about how I first fell in love with how powerful selenium can be as a tool in someone's health.

Inflammation lowers the ability to make a protein called Albumin, and when I worked at the dialysis clinic I was "graded," so to speak on the quality of Albumins patients had. I remember Dr. Z (not her name but discretions people) telling me, "She's never had a good Albumin and probably never will."

I took that as a challenge. I was going to help my patient with her inflammation and help her feel better in the process. I researched and researched and found a study that showed just three Brazil nuts a day was enough to reduce inflammation in dialysis patients.

Thyroid Supporting Nutrients

Selenium

I brought the study to my patient and said, "We're trying this." She was up for it and her daughter helped remind her every day to eat her three Brazil nuts!

Sure enough, her Albumin for three months consecutively after we started was either at or above her goal Albumin for the first time ever!!

The doctor was shocked!

I know this book is not about someone on dialysis, but this just shows how potent Selenium is as an antioxidant and how amazing food can be for us! See for yourself on the next page to learn about selenium rich foods.

What is Selenium?

Selenium is an essential trace mineral that must be obtained in the diet. It is involved in over two dozen processes in the body, some being the immune system and thyroid health.

Thyroid Supporting Nutrients

Selenium

Selenium concentration is higher in the thyroid gland than in any other organ in the body (31). Low levels of selenium have been shown to increase risk of goiters. A goiter is the abnormal enlargement of the thyroid gland and usually develops as a result of iodine deficiency or inflammation.

When selenium and iodine are present, these key nutrients protect the thyroid from potential attackers or anti-nutrients. Think of selenium and iodine as protective shields to harmful anti-nutrients. Some anti-nutrients are goitrogens and phytates.

If goitrogens are consumed frequently, and if there is a lack of selenium and iodine rich foods, this can promote goiters or abnormal growth of the thyroid. See chapter eight to learn more about goitrogens, just know that eating foods rich in selenium is extremely important because selenium protects the thyroid from goitrogenic foods. See next page for my top selenium food choices.

Selenium is a potent antioxidant, which means it's great at protecting the cells of the thyroid and other parts of the body.

Selenium Rich Foods

There is some evidence that selenium supplementation does reduce thyroid peroxidase antibody (TPO) levels in patients with autoimmune thyroiditis, Hashimoto's disease (32). However, I'm a fan of food first.

> The RDA for Selenium in adults in 55 micrograms daily!
> *One Brazil nut contains 68-91 mcg!!*

RDA: Recommend Daily Allowance

Brazil nuts are a great source of selenium.

I don't recommend eating more than three Brazil nuts a day. Too much Selenium may result in diarrhea, brittle hair or nails, or loss of appetite. Brazil nuts are easy snacking food. I will grab three Brazil nuts with a handful of blueberries for a morning snack most days. Some people with digestive issues may benefit from soaking brazil nuts in water and keep in a jar in the fridge.

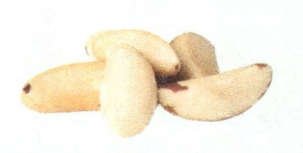

Selenium Rich Foods

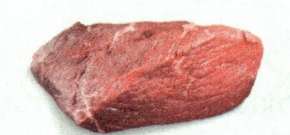

Brazil Nuts   **Grass-Fed Beef**   **Legumes**

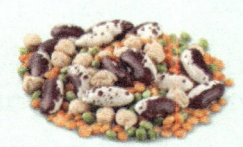

Selenium Rich Foods

Grass-fed beef is another good source of selenium and before you say, "I don't eat red meat because I'm trying to be healthier," red meat can be extremely healthy when done right. A cow that's stuck side by side to another cow, fed corn, and given antibiotics is going to have more of the pro-inflammatory fat. Those types of cows also contain more cortisol, the stress hormone, which we then ingest when we eat these types of meat. Not the best choice.

What is a good choice for beef is a cow that is free to roam around and eat the food it's meant to - grass! These cows are happier and have less cortisol. Grass fed cows aren't just stuck next to another cow, but they are free to roam in a pasture which means the type of fat is considered heart healthy because it's a more anti-inflammatory fat.

The quality of the animal's life we eat does matter, which, unfortunately, typically means the cut of meat you buy from the grocery store will be a bit more expensive.

The way to avoid big grocery bill is to limit your serving size to the size of the palm of your hand, a lot smaller than what most people consume.

Selenium Rich Foods

I grew up in Texas and worked at multiple different BBQ and other meat-heavy restaurants, where I would serve a plate that had meat on it the size of your face! That's too much but that's what is served in many places, and it's just too much.

Here's another benefit of reducing portion size of meat –allows for more space for vegetables and whole grains! This is how you don't break the bank. Brown rice is cheap, and vegetables can be cheap too.

Another great money saving tip I use is to cook with beans and lentils two to three times a week. These are in the legume family. When grocery shopping, choose mostly dried legumes so you can save even more money. Legumes are a great source of this crucial nutrient, selenium! Legumes also provide both soluble and insoluble fiber, protein, folate, potassium, iron and magnesium.

Remember to soak your legumes overnight to remove phytic acid and lectins. This just means thinking ahead is crucial. Phytic acid is a component in plants that helps keep certain nutrients in the plant, but if we eat too much phytic acid, it can impair the absorption of iron, zinc, and calcium. Soaking legumes and dumping that water out removes those anti-nutrients and leaves a food high in helpful nutrients!

Selenium Rich Foods

Tuna is not just a great source of protein and healthy fats, but it's also a good source of selenium. Eat it to help incorporate a variety of selenium rich foods. Tuna does contain mercury, which can be unhealthy for the central nervous system, especially for higher-risk populations like pregnant women's unborn children and also young children.

The body can metabolize mercury just fine in small amounts, the risk lies when high levels of mercury are consumed. I eat one can of tuna once a week, and occasionally if I didn't plan properly, two cans! Oysters are another good source of selenium but it's not a common food for many.

I'm not going to be eating it daily, but canned tuna is a quick and easy lunch and supports a healthy thyroid. I usually add an avocado oil plant-based mayonnaise, mustard (turmeric in mustard is helpful for anti-inflammatory purposes), a little black pepper, garlic powder, onion powder and diced pickles. It's easy to eat over a salad or on a sandwich made with whole wheat bread.

Selenium Rich Foods

Whole grains, like whole wheat bread, whole wheat pasta, and brown rice, are also good sources of selenium in addition to their higher fiber content.

There's an entire section dedicated to how important carbohydrates, including these selenium rich whole grains, are to the body.

Sunflower seeds are great toppers to many dishes like salads, veggie bowls, or as part of a snack. Sometimes adding these "foods as medicine" to a meal doesn't make sense before you take a bite, then you end up loving it after the second bite. Sunflower seeds also have copper, zinc, and iron - all which are thyroid friendly.

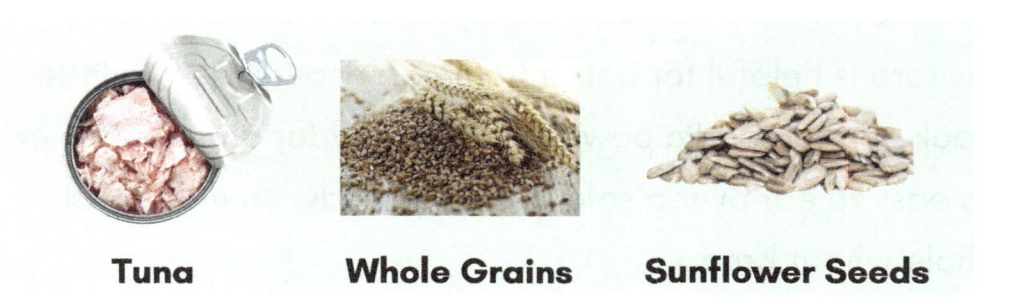

Tuna **Whole Grains** **Sunflower Seeds**

Thyroid Supporting Nutrients

Tyrosine & Iodine

The thyroid uses an amino acid, tyrosine, from the foods we eat to start making thyroid hormones (33). The thyroid gland combines tyrosine with iodine to make two main hormones, T4 and T3. Now do I want you to go out and start taking L-Tyrosine supplements, like many people do? No, tyrosine is found in many of the foods and all you have to do is start incorporating these foods into your day.

> **Caution does need to be given with tyrosine and iodine. In hyperthyroid, or Graves' disease, the body is producing too much T4 and T3. Omitting or limiting tyrosine and iodine rich foods may be helpful in this population.**

Too much iodine can suppress the thyroid gland. I never recommend my clients to take an iodine supplement, I always encourage food forms. Many people who eat a high intake of processed food likely receive too much iodine, which can worsen hypothyroidism. Incorporating more meals from home that are cooked from scratch, including foods from this guide can help ensure a proper intake of iodine from natural food sources.

Tyrosine Rich Foods

Fatty fish is a great anti-inflammatory food due to its rich source of omega 3 fatty acids. It is also a great source of the amino acid, tyrosine. Salmon is a great way to incorporate this important thyroid supporting nutrient and my favorite way to eat it is by cooking salmon on a sheet pan (see the recipe section in chapter eleven for my salmon sheet pan recipe).

Canned tuna is also an easy way to get in tyrosine, and we previously discussed how rich in selenium it is as well. I like to eat tuna once a week from a can. I know some people might say, "too much mercury," however, our bodies are designed to properly metabolize mercury out of the body in small amounts. Eating tuna plus salmon once a week is an easy way to get in your thyroid hormone supporting nutrients.

Almonds are another great source of tyrosine, in addition to protein and fiber. They're easy to add as a snack in a trail mix, as a nut butter, or as slivers on top of a salad or in green beans.

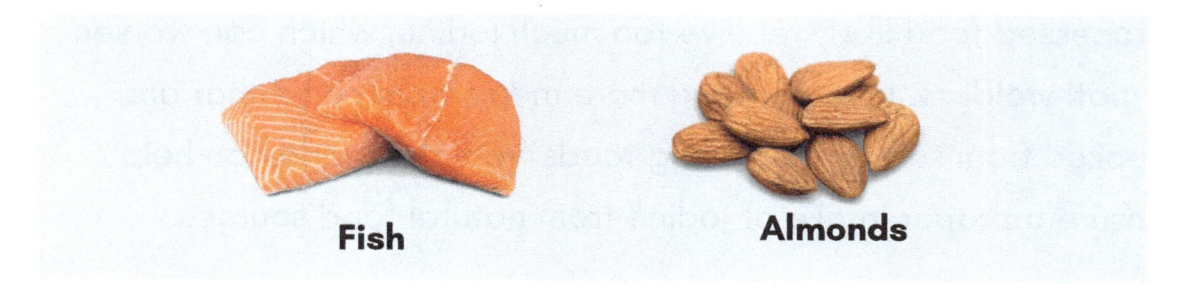

Fish   **Almonds**

Tyrosine Rich Foods

Soy is another great source of tyrosine. But the type of soy does matter. I encourage organic tofu, edamame, and soybeans. Processed soy is not going to be beneficial. My son the other day asked me to get plant based "chicken nuggets." When I looked at the ingredients ,it was extremely processed. Yes, it probably tastes good but it does not provide any benefits other than getting his belly full after eating. I expand more on soy in chapter eight when I debunk thyroid nutrition myths. Tofu is also a good source of selenium in addition to tyrosine.

Pumpkin seeds are also a great source of tyrosine. I love getting the roasted salted version of pumpkin seeds! Sometimes I just grab a handful to snack on. They're great additions to many meals and snacks. Try sprinkling the pumpkin seeds on your oatmeal, on a salad, baking into muffins, or as the crunch in a veggie rice bowl.

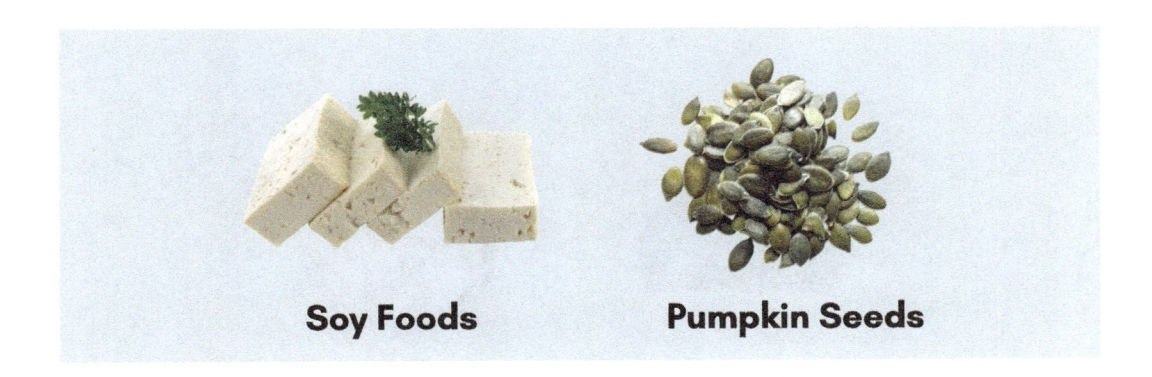

Soy Foods   **Pumpkin Seeds**

Iodine Rich Foods

Iodine is extremely important for the thyroid, but in my opinion should be only consumed in food and never in a supplement form. Supplements are not regulated and therefore it may have no iodine in it or may have two to three times the amount it says. **This can be very dangerous as too little iodine can promote hypothyroidism and too much iodine can suppress the thyroid to promote hypothyroidism.** Consistent intake of iodine in food form is best.

Eating foods that contain iodine is a safer option and you'll get other nutritional benefits by eating the food versus just a supplement.

Seaweed also contains iron and antioxidants. Seaweed can be a great tool for thyroid warriors. I used to think seaweed was gross, I tried it once, ehhhh not the best. Tried it again and liked it a little more. I kept trying it until I liked it! Now, I eat dry roasted seaweed a few times a week to support my thyroid. Try eating some dry roasted seaweed with a meal or a snack, and if you don't like it keep trying. It will grow on you.

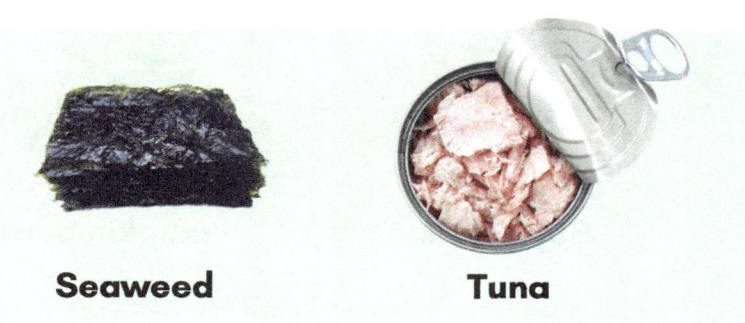

Seaweed **Tuna**

Iodine Rich Foods

Eggs are a good source of iodine, too. Unfortunately, for those that stick to only egg whites, you'll be sorely disappointed to know that you're tossing away key nutrients for your thyroid.

Iodine is found in the yolks of eggs and only accounts for a small amount of your daily need for iodine. One of my favorite ways to eat an egg is to have it fried or sunny side up on a leftover veggie bowl.

This book contains multiple veggie bowl recipes for you in the recipe section. Iodine rich foods can easily be added to your day in food form. Make sure you eat other foods that contain iodine, like whole wheat bread, yogurt, cod, and even oysters!

Yogurt is another source of iodine. I always encourage a low fat or fat free option. This allows you to add your choice of fat. Adding fats like milled flaxseed or chia seeds can increase the amounts of omega 3 fatty acids and fiber intake.

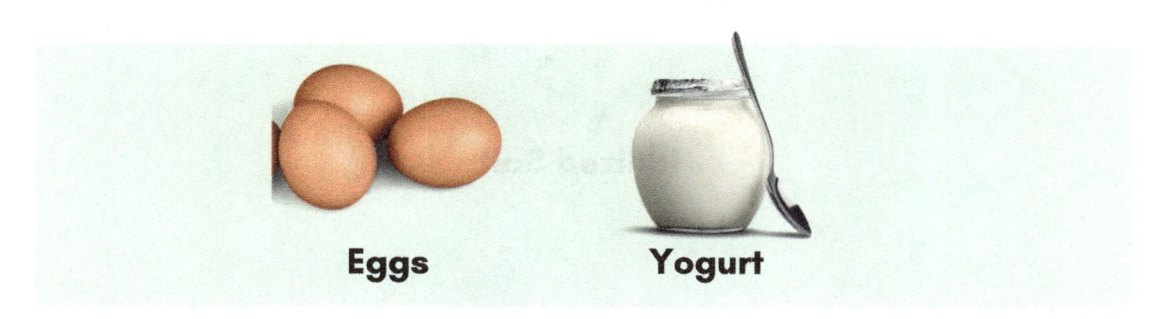

Eggs   **Yogurt**

Iodine Rich Foods

Iodized salt is an easy way to add iodine to meals! Salt is another nutrient I feel has gotten such a bad reputation because of processed foods and heart disease.

Too much salt can cause the body to hold on to more water and therefore, make more of a workload for the heart. However, we do need around 2,300 mg of sodium a day (sodium chloride is what is in table salt it).

Sodium is important for us, but the problem lies when we have too much. An easy way to get in iodized salt, without it being too much, is by reducing your intake of processed foods! When you reduce processed foods, you're also reducing potential harmful endocrine disrupting food additives. This way you have control over your iodine and can add salt to the meals you cook at home.

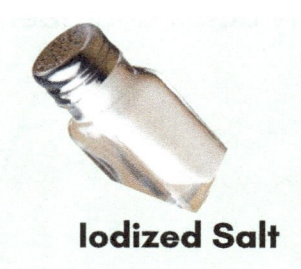

Iodized Salt

Zinc Rich Foods

Zinc plays multiple key roles in thyroid hormones by regulating TSH and influences the levels of T4 and T3 as well (34). Zinc is an essential mineral that we must eat. People that have a low zinc intake may have a loss of appetite, hair loss, or abnormalities of the nails, like white lines.

There are many different sources of zinc. Below you'll find my top four. I make grass-fed beef recipes on average once or twice a week (which means I could have it two to four days with leftovers). I eat nuts daily, beans once or twice a week, and grains a few times a week as well. See how these foods can be easily incorporated into your diet!?!

I hardly ever recommend taking a zinc supplement, as it can lead to a copper deficiency, especially if taken for longer than a two-week period.

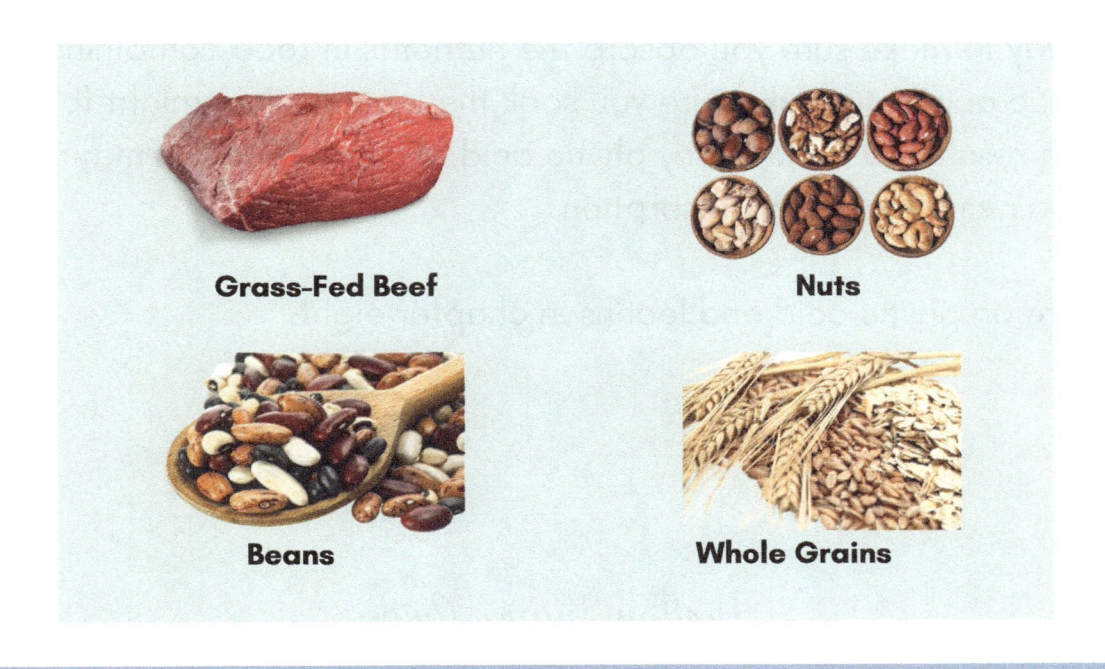

Grass-Fed Beef

Nuts

Beans

Whole Grains

Zinc Rich Foods

Grass-fed beef is more expensive, however be aware of your portion sizes. Meat serving size should not be more than the size of the palm of your hand and this portion size guidance works for kids and adults. You'll continue to read about the benefits grass-fed beef can provide you as you go through this book.

If you are a vegetarian or vegan, you can get your zinc through plants too. Nuts are an easy way to get your zinc and also provide you with healthy fats, fiber, and magnesium. Cashews are the richest sources of zinc in the nut "family," but almonds are a close second.

Legumes are also a great source of zinc. But, legumes also contain something called phytic acid which could prevent us from absorbing the zinc.

A way to make sure you absorb the nutrients in food containing phytic acid is to make sure you soak the legumes (overnight for best results) to remove any phytic acid and lectins which may impair zinc (and iron) absorption.

More on phytic acid and lectins in chapter eight.

Thyroid Supporting Nutrients

IRON

Iron is a metal that our bodies need to receive through our diets. Iron's major role in the body is to help produce hemoglobin. Hemoglobin allows oxygen to be transferred to various organs, muscles, and tissues.

Iron's also necessary in multiple steps of thyroid hormone metabolism. Iron deficiency is called anemia and can be a major factor for impaired thyroid hormone metabolism (35). Anemia by itself is exhausting and then you add thyroid exhaustion... talk about feeling depleted!

Anemia can stop or decrease TSH from being produced by the pituitary gland. If the body isn't producing enough TSH, the body is also not going to be able to produce enough T4 and T3.

Anemia can interfere with the binding of iodine to the thyroid hormones, T4 and T3. Remember T3 is the gas pedal to the car, T3 is your metabolism.

I have seen anemia happen many times, not from lack of iron in the diet but from eating too much dairy! The calcium in dairy can block iron from being absorbed.

Iron Rich Foods

Vitamin C is not just for our immune system but can also enhance iron's absorption! Eating foods high in vitamin C, like oranges, lemons, bell peppers, kiwis, and broccoli with iron rich foods helps enhance your iron intake. This a great example of how pairing foods can be helpful!

Spinach and other deep leafy green vegetables are good sources of iron. Many of the thyroid warriors I have worked with tend to also have digestive issues with severe bloating. If this is you, cook your greens for better digestion.

Legumes are another good source of iron, especially chickpeas. Legumes do contain phytic acid, so make sure to soak your beans and dump that water prior to cooking them. Phytic acid has been known to block iron absorption. Soaking plus cooking eliminates the phytic acid so you are free to absorb the iron!

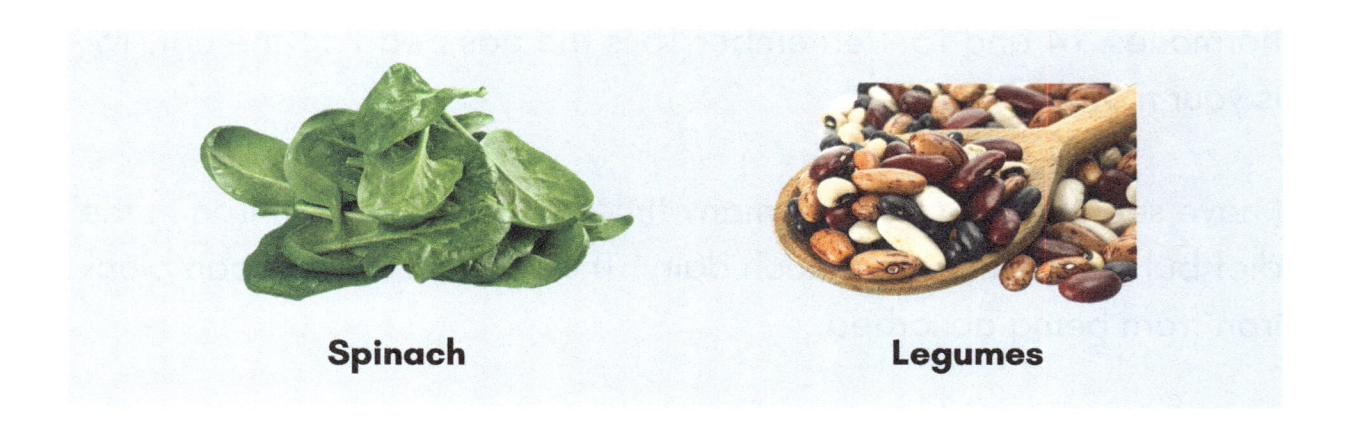

Spinach

Legumes

Iron Rich Foods

Dried apricots are a good iron source for many because they're easy travel foods. Grab a handful of apricots for a snack or cut them up on top of a salad.

Guess what food is the highest in iron? Beef! I'll keep reminding you how awesome grass-fed beef can be for a healthy thyroid. Pssssttt.... It's awesome! I typically get grass-fed beef ground, but if you can find it in cuts of meat, grab it!. I don't see it often in stores for some reason. I am starting to see more grass-fed options in things like jerky and dairy. However, dairy is high in calcium and can block iron absorption, so be aware of how often you eat it.

If you need additional iron, be careful of iron supplements as they can be constipating. There are a few other ways to add iron supplements to your foods. You can cook in cast iron skillets, as some of the iron will leach out of the pan and into the food you're cooking. I've even had a few of my clients order an iron fish to boil in water. They use that iron infused water in smoothies or in making rice, etc.

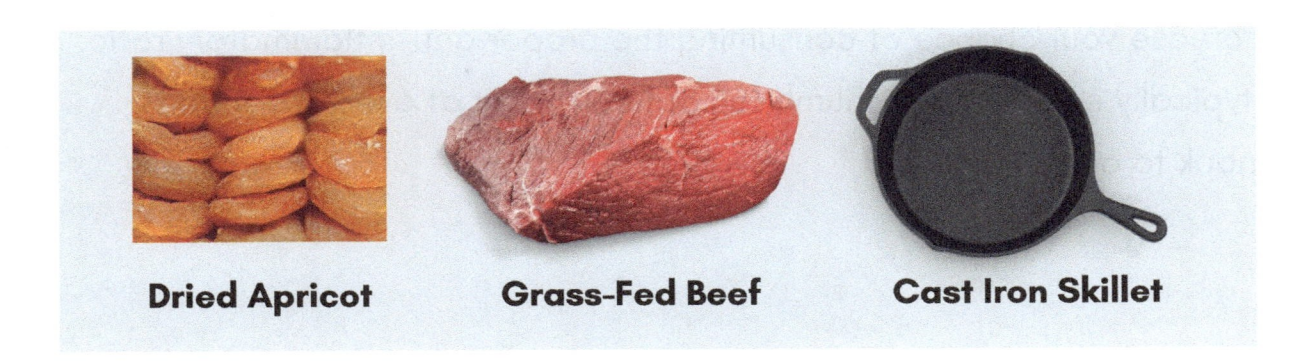

Dried Apricot   **Grass-Fed Beef**   **Cast Iron Skillet**

Thyroid Supporting Nutrients

Omega-3 Fatty Acids

Omega-3 fatty acids are one of my favorite nutrients because they're so crucial in the fight against inflammation.

Omega - fatty acids are a part of a fat group called poly-unsaturated fatty acids or PUFAs. PUFAs are made up of omega 6 and omega-3 fatty acids. *The body likes a good ratio of omega 6 to omega-3 like 2:1 or 4:1, however the western diet many people consume is upwards of 16:1.* Let that sink in. Most people eat a diet so inflammatory it's four times the amount of the recommended omega-6 intake.

We must get PUFAs from our diet, as our bodies do not make these kinds of fats. PUFAs help reduce inflammation in the body which can help protect the thyroid gland (36).

Placing the emphasis of omega-3 fatty acid containing foods will increase your chance of consuming the proper anti-inflammatory ratio. I typically encourage a thumb full of healthy fat at every meal and snack to achieve this.

Omega-3 Fatty Acid Rich Foods

The thyroid is the organ most susceptible to stress, and inflammation is a stress to the thyroid and rest of the body. I hear, "I get tired after I workout and need to rest a day" or "I'm achy and unmotivated" frequently in my practice. Reducing inflammation will help improve those exact issues.

I find that the more people incorporate healthy fats into their day, the better they feel! Hormones rely on fats to work properly, and omega 3 fatty acids help with reducing inflammation. I encourage a serving of healthy fat at every meal and snack (typically around a thumbs worth of healthy fat).

Omega-3 Fatty Acids are found in avocado, avocado oil, olives, olive oils, nuts, seeds, fatty fish like salmon, and grass-fed beef. Some can even be found in eggs and whole grains, but not a significant amount.

I've seen many people feel so much better with the introduction and consistency of these foods. However, if you're only adding a little healthy fats every once in a while, it's like tossing a pebble into a stormy body of water. Sometimes, you need to toss in a boud

Omega 3 Fatty Acid Rich Foods

I learned in school that an eighth of an avocado was an appropriate serving size, but that's when the emphasis is placed on calories. *What if you focused the amount to eat based on the demand an individual has for key nutrients?* Certain populations require a higher intake of certain nutrients and I've found that almost every thyroid client of mine benefits from a diet extremely rich in the foods pictured below.

This is partly due to the protective properties that omega-3 fatty acids give to the thyroid gland. But clients also feel better because omega-3 fatty acids improve their overall hormone health, help with anxiety reduction, and even for some people ease pain.

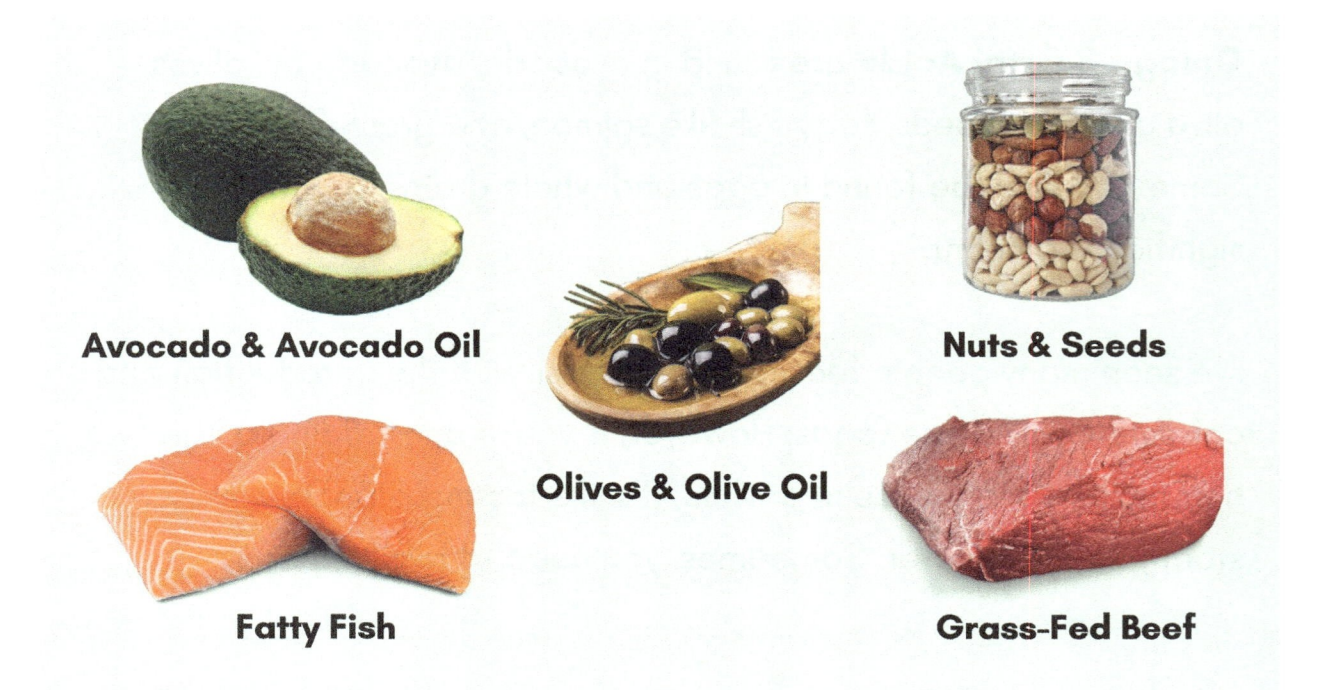

Avocado & Avocado Oil

Olives & Olive Oil

Nuts & Seeds

Fatty Fish

Grass-Fed Beef

Omega 3 Fatty Acid Rich Foods

Avocados are a great source of omega-3 fatty acids. They are also a great source of fiber and magnesium. I've been mentioning magnesium but haven't quite elaborated yet.

Magnesium has over 300 different roles in the body and for the body to work properly, a diet rich in magnesium is helpful. Many of the omega-3 fatty acid rich foods are also a good source of magnesium. Both omega-3 fatty acids and magnesium play a role in stress and anxiety reduction. This is just another reason to always rely on food for nutrition over supplements.

Other foods high in magnesium include: pumpkin seeds, chia seeds, almonds, cashews, cooked spinach, and black beans. Notice that most these foods also contain beneficial omega-3 fatty acids.

With that said, I still take a fish oil supplement daily because I don't eat fish more than once or twice a week.

We've discussed salmon before because of it's tyrosine content and how helpful it is for making T4 and T3 hormones. Salmon is one of the richest sources of omega-3 fatty acids in fish. It should be wild caught for best quality however, this does make salmon more expensive. Portion sizes matter, especially with higher quality protein sources.

Omega 3 Fatty Acid Rich Foods

Try going to a large wholesale store like Costco or Sam's Club to buy in bulk. Freeze portioned out servings. It's easier to cut fresh than cutting frozen fish. If able, try to factor it in the grocery bill once a week.

I like to keep meal planning cheap and olives can be a great, inexpensive way to get in healthy fats. I enjoy incorporating olives on top of a veggie bowl, on pastas, and as a part of my snack.

Random snacks like olives, fruit, and a little piece of cheese are delicious. Speaking of random snacks, nuts are my number one go to snack food.

All nuts are not created equally. Peanut butter seems to be such the craze but, in reality, it doesn't match up to other nuts because its omega-3 fatty acid content is minimal. But walnuts, WOW! Walnuts are my favorite nut, aside from Brazil nuts, due to their rich nutrient content.

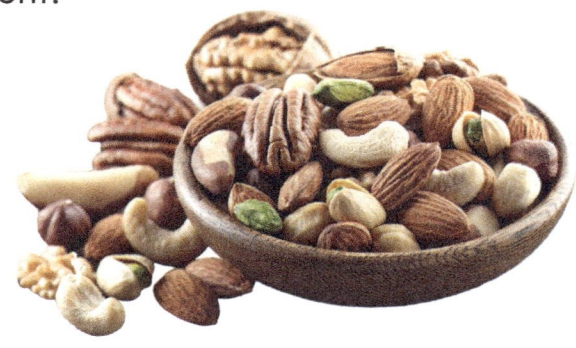

Omega-3 Fatty Acid Rich Foods

Walnuts are shaped like the brain for a reason. Walnuts contain the highest concentration of DHA, which is a type of omega-3 fatty acid. DHA is an important component of every cell in the body. It's essential for brain development and function, as it may affect the speed and quality of communication between nerve cells. DHA is also important for eye health and may reduce risk factors for many health diseases.

Later, you'll learn how stress and anxiety are related to thyroid health in more depth, but know now that the more you are stressed or have anxiety the higher demand you have for omega-3 fatty acids. Eating a diet rich in omega-3 fatty acids may help improve your moods, which will lessen the stress on the thyroid.

I typically aim for half a cup of nuts a day plus two to three tablespoons of seeds to help with my healthy fat intake! Sheet pan salmon meals are fast and easy, with salmon being rich in DHA and EPA. Eating meals like chili, homemade burgers, or sweet potato tacos- anything with grass-fed beef is a great way to achieve this too.

Caution to people who are on blood thinners or have a clotting disorder. Increasing omega-3 fatty acids will thin the blood some, which is part of the reason why it's so heart healthy. Please speak to your doctor or dietitian if you are someone at risk for bleeds.

Thyroid Supporting Nutrients

B-Vitamins

B-vitamins are necessary as the body uses them to get or make energy from food. They also help form red blood cells. Remember discussing how anemia or low iron can perpetuate hypothyroidism? This is how B-vitamins, particularly low B-vitamins, may have a negative impact on the thyroid.

40% of people that are diagnosed with hypothyroidism are also vitamin B12 deficient (37). I've also noticed in my practice that many people with thyroid disorders also have the MTHFR gene mutation. A MTHFR gene mutation means the body is unable to take B-vitamins and convert them to their active form (which tends to lead to elevated homocysteine levels...hello allergies... and a folate or B12 deficiency also known as megaloblastic anemia).

Upwards of 55% of people with European descent have the MTHFR gene mutation. I'm of this descent and take a methylated B complex daily. These vitamins are easy to find as it says methylcobalamin instead of cyanocobalamin for B12 component.

It may be helpful to get a lab work up if you think you may be at risk. This is a great discussion to have with your doctor.

B-Vitamin Rich Foods

B-vitamins are found in many different foods; however, B12 is mainly found in animal sources. Vegetarians or vegans may require close monitoring of B12 levels and may need a supplement.

Organ meats are the highest in B12. Go for it if you can eat them, I can't. I'm sharing the foods high in B-vitamins that are more commonly consumed.

Beets are a great source of B-vitamins and also glutathione. Beets are a flavor that I am still getting used to. Yes, a dietitian doesn't always like all the foods! I'm currently eating beets in their fermented form and adding a 100% beet juice into smoothies.

Fish is a great source of B12, especially sardines! Salmon is a good source for your B-vitamins and grass-fed beef as well. Can you tell which foods you should be eating more often now? Start rotating in grass-fed beef and salmon into your weekly meal plan.

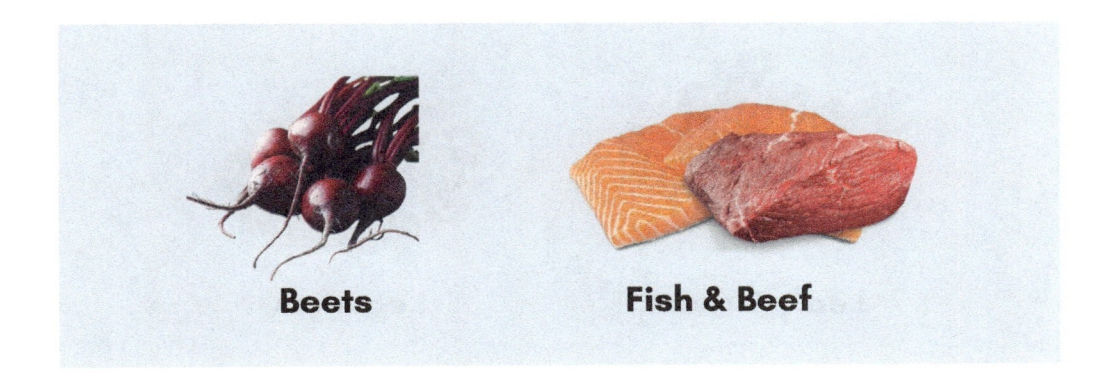

Beets   **Fish & Beef**

B-Vitamin Rich Foods

Green leafy veggies are also a good source of folate, another important B-vitamin. I personally like spinach the best for daily use, but I love to explore other options like arugula because it has a mustardy taste or kale in soup because it holds up well.

Improve the taste of your meals by using the color wheel for guidance. Green leafy vegetables tend to be more bitter. Pair those bitter flavors with sweeter ones found opposite green on the color wheel with reds, oranges, and yellow vegetables.

People who have digestive issues may benefit from cooking their greens versus eating them raw.

Legumes are a good source of B-vitamins, zinc, iron, and protein. I like to use beans as part of my breakfast when I make a sweet potato taco. I had to share the recipe with you, so check it out in the recipe section.

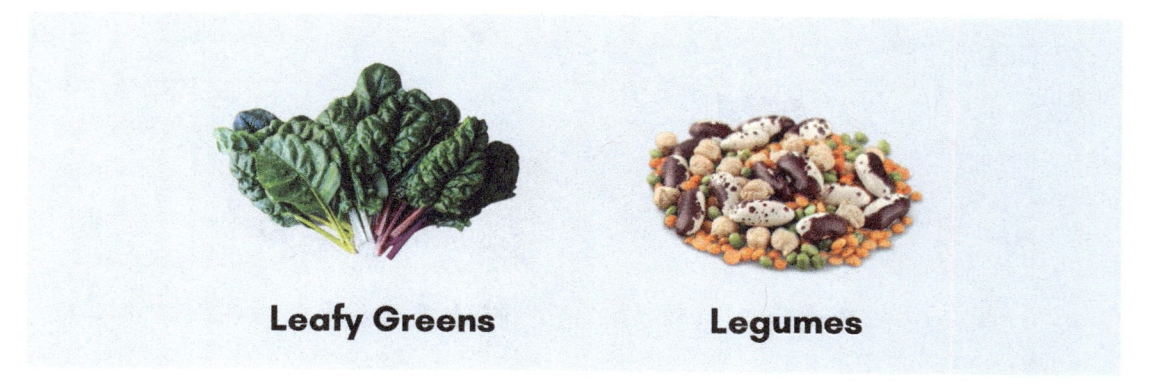

Leafy Greens **Legumes**

Thyroid Supporting Nutrients

Carbohydrates

Carbohydrates are our bodies preferred energy source. Around 60% of our calories should be coming from carbohydrates (better known as carbs). I know!

Your jaw is probably on the ground, I'll wait while you pick it up! Yes 60% of our daily calories can come from carbs. Many people associate all carbs as bad but in reality it's the processed ones that give us the most trouble.

The problem is carbs have gotten a bad reputation over the years. Many people I encounter have once or are currently reducing their carb intake in an attempt to lose weight or decrease blood sugars.

When carb intake is drastically reduced, conversion of T3 from T4 declines (38). This shows us that the body needs steady blood glucose levels to have readily available tools for the thyroid to do its job.

Carbohydrates

The goal is to keep a steady intake of carbohydrates throughout the day.

We achieve this by **eating mostly complex carbohydrates** (basically think when fiber is present) and those **carbs are paired with a protein or fat source.** Aim to **eat within 2 hours of waking up** (even if you can only eat a handful of berries and some walnuts or seeds- that's a great start towards supporting your metabolism/thyroid), **eating consistently throughout the day**, and **minimizing refined sugars**.

> **Case Study**: A client came to me suffering from fatigue and exhaustion. She was drinking a protein shake before working out, only a coffee after working out, and would eat low carb lunches and dinners. She started incorporating berries into her shake, having a carb with a protein for post-workout meal, adding quinoa to her salads. Immediately, she started having more energy, no longer crashing at 2pm, and started feeling better! Carbohydrates are necessary in the diet.

Carbohydrates

Carbohydrates empty from the stomach faster than protein or fats. This is why it's important to pair your carbs with a protein or fat. This can be as simple as a handful of nuts and berries.

This is an important step to remember because if you eat carbs by themselves, it can increase your blood glucose levels. When you just eat carbs the stomach will empty it out fast and the carbs will be absorbed into the blood stream fast. This can lead to inflammation, amongst other things, and unfortunately, the thyroid is easily affected by inflammation.

You might be wondering how the heck you're going to eat carbs but not raise your blood sugars and cause inflammation!?!

The answer is that you must eat carbohydrates with a fat and/or protein source AND you must eat three meals a day. I'm talking to you, breakfast or lunch skipper.

Skipping meals, or avoiding carbs at meals, can have a negative effect on the blood sugars. The habit of skipping meals is something that causes a lot of difficulties in the body: blood sugar dysregulation, hormones are affected, and energy levels are zapped.

Carbohydrates

Pair your food!

Eating nuts or nut butters, seeds, grass-fed beef jerky, and avocado- to name a few options- with your carbohydrate source will decrease the release of glucose into the bloodstream by slowing the release of food out of the stomach. This will have a ripple effect on the body. This is why I love the plate method for guidance in a meal This is how you maximize your nutrients – just eat a colorful meal or snack! See recipes for how I pair the snack options and meals in chapter eleven.

The quality of carbs matters. I haven't been talking about processed crackers, chips, and cakes, even though they do have their time and place in a healthy lifestyle, I'm talking about complex carbs! "Complex carbs" simply mean they have fiber in them! Good source of complex carbohydrates include, but are not limited to:

Oats, quinoa, sweet potato, berries, wild rice, squash, apples, pears, potatoes, bananas, kiwi, beets, turmeric, beans, papaya, tomato, and carrot.

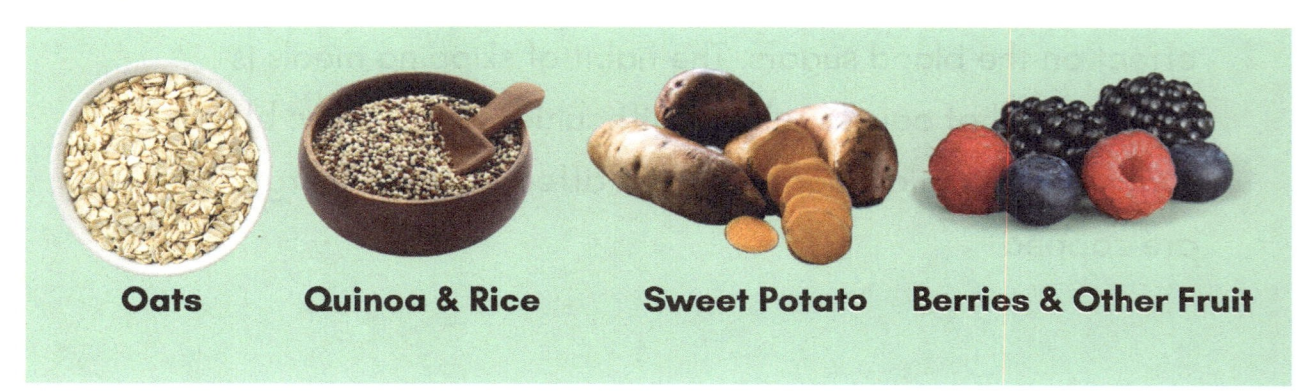

Oats **Quinoa & Rice** **Sweet Potato** **Berries & Other Fruit**

Thyroid Supporting Nutrients

COPPER

Copper is a trace element, important for the function of many cellular enzymes (39). One of those being with the thyroid hormone, T4. Copper stimulates the production of thyroxine T4 and prevents overabsorption of T4 in the blood cells by controlling the body's calcium levels (40).

Below you'll find the copper rich foods I like to eat. I aim to eat some on a daily basis and some weekly; however, I do try to get in as much as I can.

I, personally, eat avocado almost daily, cashews a few times a week, quinoa or lentils once a week. I don't like the taste of almonds, so I go for cashews, just a personal preference. You can see ways to incorporate some of these foods into your diet with the recipes provided in chapter eleven.

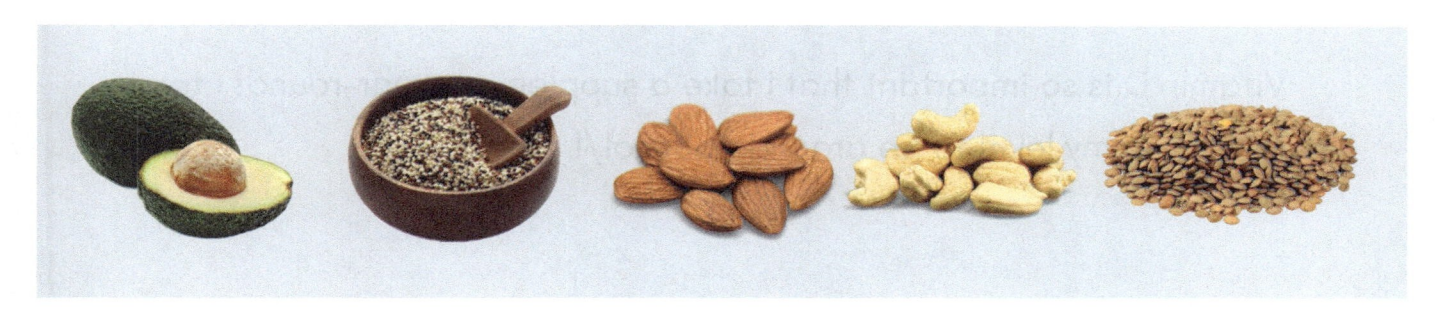

Thyroid Supporting Nutrients

Vitamin D

Vitamin D deficiency is extremely common and with the recent pandemic in 2020, I saw an increase in low vitamin D levels in many of my clients. If you're not getting outside to receive the sunlight your body needs, immune health suffers tremendously. Low vitamin D levels can make you feel tired, run down, impair certain hormone functions, and decreases immune function.

Studies shows that vitamin D are significantly lower in hypothyroid patients than in controls (41). It is well documented that vitamin D levels tend to be lower in women than in men.

Maintaining good vitamin D levels is complex. I've seen people who work outside for a living and still have low levels of vitamin D. I see people that go outside frequently each day and who are vitamin D deficient. I notice a strong correlation in my practice with people who have autoimmune diseases and low vitamin D levels .

Vitamin D is so important that I take a supplement year-round! I try to aim for my level to be around 60 nmol/L (7).

Thyroid Supporting Nutrients

Vitamin D

> **Vitamin D Case Study**: One of my clients worked 12-hour shifts, 5 days a week. They went to work before the sun came up and was home from work after the sun went down. This person only saw the sun on the weekend and it just wasn't enough. They were getting sick often, really run down, crying a lot, were depressed, and getting cold sores frequently.

I had a suspicion their vitamin D level was low. Once the labs came back at 23 (optimal levels are around 60-80 nmol/L) I knew they needed to get started on vitamin D supplement right away. The RDA is what is recommend for the average American and is set at 400 IU. However, when a level is low, a higher intake of vitamin D is necessary.

She started taking 5,000 IU of vitamin D every morning.

Once levels were up in the 40s, the individual started feeling better but we still maintained the higher dose of vitamin D until 60 nmol/L was achieved. Vitamin D can be toxic to the body, so once her optimal level was achieved I dropped her down to a maintenance dose.

Water

It's difficult for so many because it doesn't taste like much. I find for many people who are used to drinking sugary beverages, that water isn't exciting for them. Infusing water can be a great way to increase the palatability. For some people drinking water is difficult because they don't remember to drink it. Putting your cup on your desk or in your car can help remind you to drink more.

What if I told you that just a 2% decrease in body water can cause brain fog? Would that motivate you to drink more?

The National Academies of Science, Engineering and Medicine recommends that men drink about 3.7 liters (about 125 ounces) a day and women drink 2.7 liters (about 91 ounces) a day. Now, this does vary based on activity level and health (like diarrhea). Certain foods count as water intake. Oranges, melons, pineapples, and grapefruits are high water foods.

I find that people drink more water when they have a fun cup to drink out of and when they use a straw. Set reminders on your phone if you have to. Water is that important, and it's important that you're drinking water that's been filtered enough to remove medications and endocrine disruptors.

Water

Water is extremely helpful for gut health, for cognitive function, lubrication, and so much more. Many people with thyroid disorders get scared to drink city waters because of one ingredient, fluoride. City water tends to have fluoride added to protect people's teeth from tooth decay and should contain around 0.70 mg of fluoride per liter of water, according to the state of California (42). Check your state water board for regulations near you.

High fluoride exposure (markedly greater than in the water supply) has been associated with hypothyroidism, especially in the setting of iodine deficiency (43). However, fluoride levels are monitored. I looked up my city's water report and it's measuring right at 0.70 mg/L.

With that said, do I drink the city's tap water? I don't. We use water that's been through reverse osmosis and other filters. We do this because city water tends to have medications in the water and endocrine disruptors like, phthalates (remember chapter four and lifestyle factors that affect the thyroid). Don't let this scare you, water is crucial for us.

I feel like everyone knows the importance of drinking water, so why is it so difficult for so many?

Water

It's difficult for so many because it doesn't taste like much. I find for many people who are used to drinking sugary beverages, that water isn't exciting for them. Infusing water can be a great way to increase the palatability. For some people drinking water is difficult because they don't remember to drink it. Putting your cup on your desk or in your car can help remind you to drink more.

What if I told you that just a 2% decrease in body water can cause brain fog? Would that motivate you to drink more?

The National Academies of Science, Engineering and Medicine recommends that men drink about 3.7 liters (about 125 ounces) a day and women drink 2.7 liters (about 91 ounces) a day. Now, this does vary based on activity level and health (like diarrhea). Certain foods count as water intake. Oranges, melons, pineapples, and grapefruits are high water foods.

I find that people drink more water when they have a fun cup to drink out of and when they use a straw. Set reminders on your phone if you have to. Water is that important, and it's important that you're drinking water that's been filtered enough to remove medications and endocrine disruptors.

Chapter Eight

Nutrition Confusion

One thing that I hear all the time from people I work with is how confusing the thyroid diet is! I have to agree with them because there are so many different recommendations made by so many different people. The scary part is some of these recommendations are coming from people who have no nutrition background or science degrees.

I see this happen a lot on social media, with celebrities promoting quick fixes and even between friends and family. Just because a trend or a person is popular, does not mean their method is safe and effective!

Take the keto diet trend. When someone puts their body into ketosis, the body is using it's back up energy source. Many people will claim they've lost weight on the keto diet, but most of the weight loss is water. Also, there are many negative affects ketosis causes the body, including digestive issues (dysbiosis, bloating, constipation, pain/discomfort), increased cholesterol, decreased thyroid function, and abnormal hormone health. This is why I had an entire section dedicated to carbohydrates. I want you to understand the importance of them!!

Over the next few pages, we're going to discuss some other thyroid nutrition myths. Hopefully, you will start to see that you DON'T have to restrict or remove foods from your diet to keep your thyroid healthy!

Nutrition Thyroid Myths

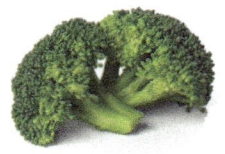

GOITROGENS

Goitrogens are substances that disrupt the production of thyroid hormones by interfering with iodine uptake in the thyroid gland. This triggers the pituitary to release thyroid-stimulating hormone, which then promotes the growth of thyroid tissue, eventually leading to goiter. Naturally occurring goitrogens are found in legumes, plants, cabbage, cauliflower broccoli, turnip, cassava root, and even in amiodarone (heart medication) and, lithium (psychiatric medication) (44).

However, I eat these foods all the time. (Gasp from the reader, I know!)

You need A LOT of goitrogens to have a negative impact on the thyroid. Someone would need to eat 194 mol of goitrogens to decrease uptake of iodine. A 100-gram serving of broccoli contains 10mol of goitrogens. This means that you would need to eat over 4 pounds of broccoli per day, every day, to inhibit the thyroid (45).

Foods like broccoli, cauliflower, spinach, kale, and cabbage all have anti-cancer properties, so eating them is more beneficial than avoiding them.

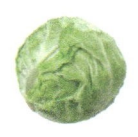

Nutrition Thyroid Myths

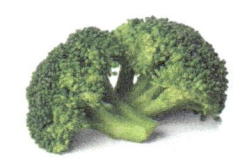

GOITROGENS

So, what's the best way for us health warriors to eat these goitrogen containing foods?

Goitrogens are actually destroyed by cooking (45). Cooking goitrogen rich foods will allow you to incorporate them into your diet, which is important due to their fiber and cancer fighting properties. Roasting them in the oven is my favorite way to eat them! 400 - 425°F with a little avocado oil drizzle, plus garlic powder, for 25 minutes to make an easy delicious meal.

Who is at risk for having goitrogen foods impacting their thyroid?

People with suboptimal intake of selenium and iodine may be negatively impacted by goitrogens. Selenium is such a potent antioxidant that protects the thyroid gland. Without adequate amounts of selenium, the thyroid is open to being harmed.

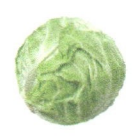

Nutrition Thyroid Myths

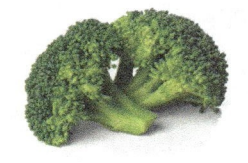

GOITROGENS

As you read this Healthy Thyroid Guide, I hope you notice that including a variety of different foods in your diet helps your body receive the nutrients it needs. Variety is also important because some foods enhance the nutrients in other foods.

For example, adding citrus to iron-rich food helps the iron be absorbed due to the citrus' vitamin C. And, bringing it back to goitrogens, eating tuna or seaweed, iodine rich foods, with Brazil nuts, rich in selenium, daily allows you to enjoy roasted broccoli, stews with cooked cabbage, and cooked lentils without needing to overthink or worry!

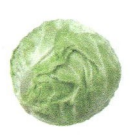

Nutrition Thyroid Myths

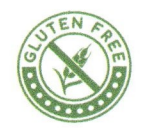

GLUTEN FREE IS THE ONLY WAY

Gluten is a protein found in wheat, barely, and rye. I eat it most days without a problem; however, many people do feel better removing gluten from their diet. This can be due to a few reasons. First, many people are fiber deficient and gluten containing foods in their natural form contain fiber. If your digestion is not used to fiber, you may not have enough of the beneficial bacteria to help break it down. If you don't have enough beneficial bacteria to break down the fiber, you may experience some intestinal discomfort.

The second reason people may feel better after removing gluten is because their gut wall integrity is suffering. This means instead of an impenetrable, brick and mortar gut wall, the gut wall is like a chain link fence allowing partially digested food through. As you can imagine, this may be the problem.

I don't think it's necessary for everyone to remove gluten from their diet, just those that are noticing some issues. When gut wall repair is complete, re-introduction of these foods can happen and will likely be tolerated.

I frequently see the correlation of gluten intolerance to poor gut health and stress. Tackle stress along side gut repair, and many foods that were thought to be problems are no longer an issue.

Nutrition Thyroid Myths

DAIRY

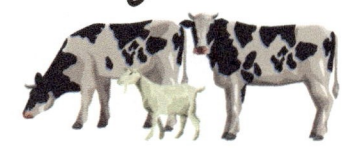

Most dairy in the stores are higher in omega-6 fatty acids. The cows who produce this are placed side by side with other cows. They don't get to move around much.

Without much movement in the cows' lives, the type of fat that's in dairy is saturated fat. Saturated fats have been associated with heart disease and inflammatory disorders. These cows also eat mostly grains or corn, which their bodies do not digest well. Many cows will need antibiotics due to mastitis or infections because they live too close to other cows (more like crammed in like sardines) and are improperly fed.

Grass-fed dairy sources are going to be the best dairy option. Grass-fed cows are happier cows, which means a better fat profile. Grass-fed cows are allowed to eat grass, which is easily digestible and results in less inflammation and infections. Grass-fed cows also have more omega-3 fatty acids and less omega-6 fatty acids to allow for a healthier fat profile (46).

Dairy by itself is not inflammatory but the cumulative intake of more omega-6 fatty containing foods compared to omega-3 fatty acids is.

Nutrition Thyroid Myths

DAIRY

I do find it difficult to find grass-fed dairy and typically just opt for very small amounts of cheese maybe once or twice a week, and dairy free milk most of the time. Moral of story: limit your dairy.

Are dairy milk alternatives beneficial?

I personally drink almond milk; however, I enjoy oat and macadamia nut milk a lot as well. Dairy milk alternatives are not better than dairy or do they provide tons of beneficial nutrition. In fact, they're mostly water. Dairy milk alternatives do have added sugars for taste, so make sure to choose the lowest added sugar containing dairy milk alternative.

The reason why I drink my turmeric latte every morning with almond milk is because it allows room in my diet to eat cheese. I love cheese and don't want to eliminate cheese just because it has inflammatory properties. I strongly believe all foods fit into a healthy lifestyle. The key is to make sure these pro-inflammatory foods are in small amounts and aren't at most of your meals.

Nutrition Thyroid Myths

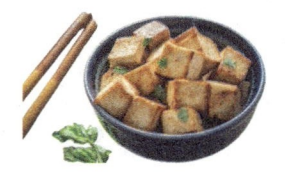

SOY

Soy has been said to be harmful to the thyroid; however, if you have an adequate amount of iodine in your body, soy has no impact on the thyroid at all.

A study reviewed 14 trials in which the effects of soy foods or isoflavones on at least one measure of thyroid function was assessed in presumably healthy subjects. Eight involved women only, four involved men only, and two both men and women. With only one exception, either no effects or only very modest changes were noted in these trials. Collectively the findings provide little evidence that in euthyroid (*having a normally functioning thyroid gland*), individuals with adequate iodine in their blood, soy foods, or isoflavones, adversely affect thyroid function (47).

What this is saying is that if you eat a variety of foods that contain iodine, (like seaweed, iodized salt, eggs, and grass-fed beef), eating soy food does not have a negative impact on the thyroid gland. This is why it's so important to eat thyroid supporting foods daily. See chapter seven for examples of thyroid supporting foods.

Nutrition Thyroid Myths
SOY

Soy has been shown to be cardiovascular protective, too! I'm a fan of organic soy as it is a good source of tyrosine, a key nutrient in having optimal thyroid hormones.

I encourage organic soy, because you want to avoid foods sprayed with potentially harmful chemicals like glyphosate.

Soy has many beneficial claims to it, like warding off osteoporosis, being good for heart health, and even preventing breast cancer. However, one must note the importance of whole soy foods vs processed soy foods.

Eat whole soy foods

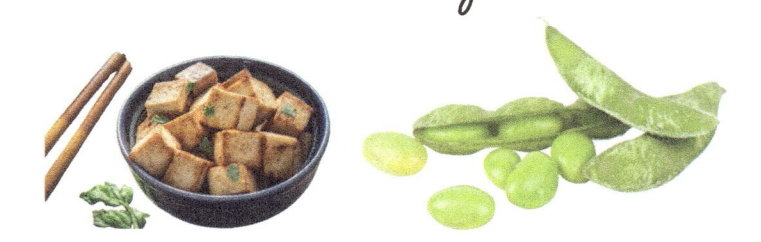

Minimize processed soy foods

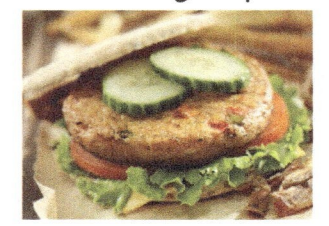

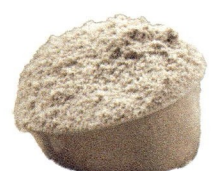

soy protein powders

Nutrition Thyroid Myths

LECTINS

Lectins are found in all plants, but raw legumes (beans, lentils, peas, soybeans, peanuts) and whole grains like wheat contain the highest amounts of lectins. Lectins have been called an "anti-nutrient" because they can interfere with the absorption of other nutrients like zinc, iron, calcium, and phosphorus. But are they really that bad for us?

Lectins are proteins that bind to carbohydrates. The same features that lectins use to defend plants in nature may cause problems during human digestion and may interfere with absorption of key nutrients like iron and zinc.

Consuming foods high in lectin is extremely rare because these foods that have the highest concentration in their raw forms are very rarely consumed raw. Beans, lentils, peas, and whole grains are usually consumed after they've been cooked.

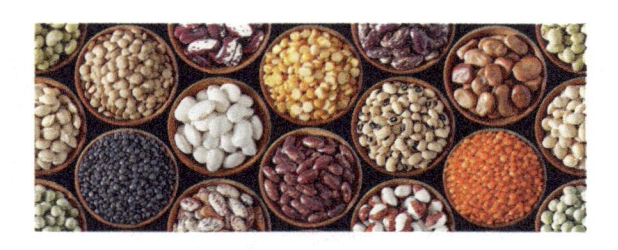

Nutrition Thyroid Myths

LECTINS

How do we typically cook these foods? You're right, by boiling them! Boiling lectins or using high heat denatures these lectin proteins and that means the foods are of no harm. This does mean low heat, or a slow cooker won't break down the lectins, so high-heat is a must. High-heat is also used to make canned beans, as a result they are also low in lectins.

Lectins can act as an antioxidant, which protects cells from damage caused by free radicals. They also slow down digestion and the absorption of carbohydrates, which may prevent sharp rises in blood sugar and high insulin levels (48)

In many large population studies, lectin-containing foods like legumes, whole grains, and nuts are associated with lower rates of cardiovascular disease, weight gain, and type 2 diabetes. These foods are rich sources of B vitamins, protein, fiber, minerals, and healthy fats.

The benefits of eating these foods outweigh their risk.

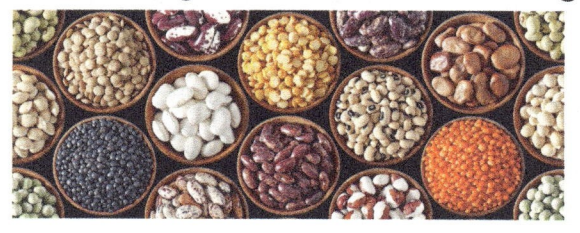

Thyroid Health Vegan or Vegetarian

In this book, you've read a lot on how beneficial grass-fed beef is and how helpful fatty fish can be for thyroid warriors. However, what if you're a vegan or vegetarian? Can this population have a healthy thyroid, even without these foods?

The answer is yes; however, attention to the person's B12 and iron status. Animal sources of proteins contain more bioavailable sources of iron and vitamin B12. This means that, as humans, we absorb these nutrients better than if they were from a plant source. If we had 10mg of iron from both animal sources and plant sources, our bodies would absorb about 3mg from the animal and only up to 1mg from plants (49).

As discussed in chapter seven, iron deficiency can prevent the body from making the proper thyroid hormones. If you think you may be deficient, it's a good idea to talk to your doctor or dietitian about your iron status so the proper labs are obtained and diet changes and/or supplementation can happen. Plant based iron sources are apricots, chickpeas, legumes, and deep green leafy vegetables.

Vitamin B12 is a crucial vitamin as it helps with the nervous system and energy. B12 is absorbed in the small intestine using something called the intrinsic factor. As we age, the intrinsic factor has been shown to migrate and even go away. People who don't eat meat are at a higher risk of this happening. Plant based sources of B12 include seaweed, nutritional yeast, tempeh, mushrooms, and fortified dairy free milks.

Chapter Nine

How to Eat for Your Thyroid

How to eat for your thyroid

Step One
Eat an Anti-Inflammatory Diet.

- **Meals should follow the Plate Method** (see two pages from now).
    - Fill half of your plate with vegetables, a quarter of your plate with protein, a quarter of your plate carbs, and a thumbs worth of healthy fat. This method puts the emphasis on portion control, color, and includes anti-inflammatory healthy fats.

- **Snacks should include a complex carbohydrate paired with a protein and/or fat.** An example of this is a piece of fruit or half cup of berries paired with a handful of nuts or hard boiled egg. Another great snack is hummus and carrots.

- **Incorporate foods that support inflammation reduction** (find my top anti-inflammatory foods in three pages)

How to eat for your thyroid

Step One
Eat an Anti-Inflammatory Diet.

- **Choose your soul food comfort level: 80/20 or 90/10**
  - Every person has a different relationship with food. Some people have a past of eating disorders, and some people have dieted every year of their adult lives. Either of which may require more flexibility in the foods they eat. Some people have a great relationship with food and can do a month or two of being really focused on the anti-inflammatory diet. *Eating food for the soul simply means you're not judging the food or yourself, but eating it because it fills up your soul*! It could be a brunch with your besties or a sporadic soft serve with the kids. Life happens, enjoy the moment.

  - 80/20: 80% of the time you're eating foods that are helpful and make you feel good and 20% of the time you're eating foods that fill up your soul. Note some days may look more like 70/30 and some 90/10... *Give yourself grace and keep asking, "Is this food or meal making me feel good?" If the answer is yes, eat that more often*!

  - 90/10: 90% of the time you're eating foods that make you feel good & 10% of the time it feeds your soul.

Portion Sizes Matter

When eating healthy, it's important to keep in mind your portion sizes.

Plate Method: YES

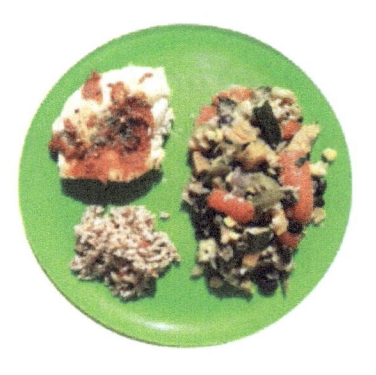

Half the plate should be your vegetables
Fourth of the plate should be protein
Fourth of the plate should be grains

What NOT to do

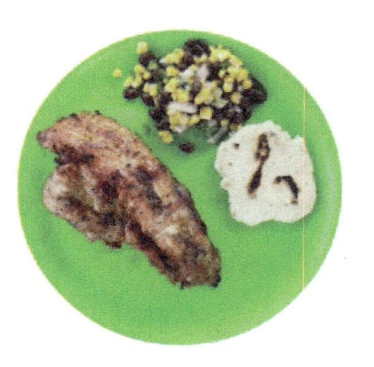

Half of this plate is meat instead of vegetables.

Basic Guidelines

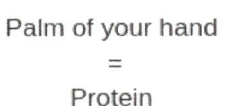

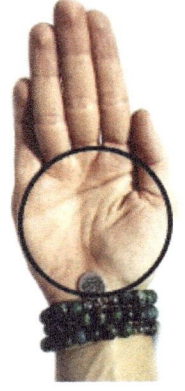

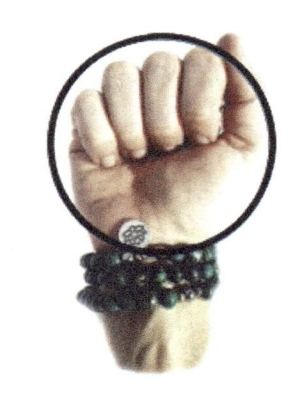

Palm of your hand
=
Protein

Fist
=
Vegetables

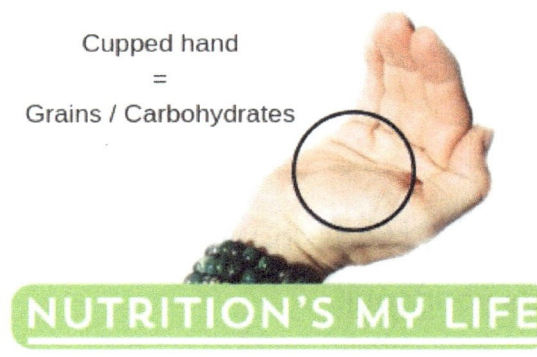

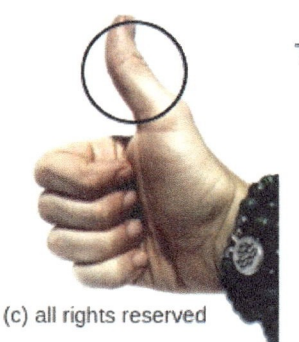

Cupped hand
=
Grains / Carbohydrates

Thumb
=
Fat

NUTRITION'S MY LIFE

(c) all rights reserved

Anti-Inflammatory Foods

Step One: First step is decreasing the processed foods in your diet.

Step Two: Start adding the following foods to your diet. Remember to increase your water intake, as you're increasing your fiber intake too!

Protein

- Air chilled chicken (no antibiotics- no added hormones)
- Grass-fed beef
- Wild caught fish (fatty fish - salmon, trout, cod, tuna, tilapia)
- Pasture raised eggs (organic - no antibiotics - no added hormones)

Vegetables

- Green leafy vegetables (spinach, kale, collards, Swiss chard, bok choy), green bell peppers, broccoli, brussels sprouts
- Tomatoes, red bell peppers
- Onion, garlic, celery
- Sweet potatoes, butternut squash, yellow/orange bell peppers, carrots

Grains

- Oatmeal
- Quinoa, freekeh, amaranth, black rice
- Brown rice
- Buckwheat, bulgur

Fats

- Olives
- Oils: avocado, olive, & sparingly use coconut
- Grass-fed butter
- Unsalted nuts and seeds (to include milled flaxseed and chia seeds as well)
- Avocado
- Hummus made with olive oil
- Fatty fish

Fruit

- Blueberry, blackberry, strawberries, raspberries
- Cherries
- Oranges and grapefruit
- Pineapple
- Papaya

Other

- Spices (cinnamon, turmeric, cardamom, ginger, black pepper)
- Bone broth
- Fresh herbs (oregano, parsley, basil, cilantro, rosemary, thyme)

Disclaimer: There are more anti-inflammatory foods than listed here, however eating from each of these groups daily will assist with reducing inflammation in the body

How to eat for your thyroid

Step One
Eat an anti-inflammatory diet.

- Reduce foods that promote inflammation.
    - Inflammatory foods include highly processed foods, fried foods, refined sugars, animal sources that are not grass-fed or pasture-raised, and large amounts of dairy.
    - Remember I said reduce. If you get quality ingredients, foods like ice cream occasionally fit into an anti-inflammatory diet.

Count your chemicals, not your calories.

- Remove foods that are causing you trouble
    - If you notice a certain food is causing you trouble, remove it for a while. Then do a trial run with reintroducing the food after some healing has occurred. Keep in mind gut healing can take up to nine months.

How to eat for your thyroid

Step Two
Add Thyroid Supporting Foods

- Start adding foods that support the thyroid into your anti-inflammatory meals. Remember reading about thyroid supporting nutrients in chapter seven? Aim to incorporate these key nutrients into your day.
    - See following page for a list of thyroid supporting foods.

Thyroid Supporting Foods

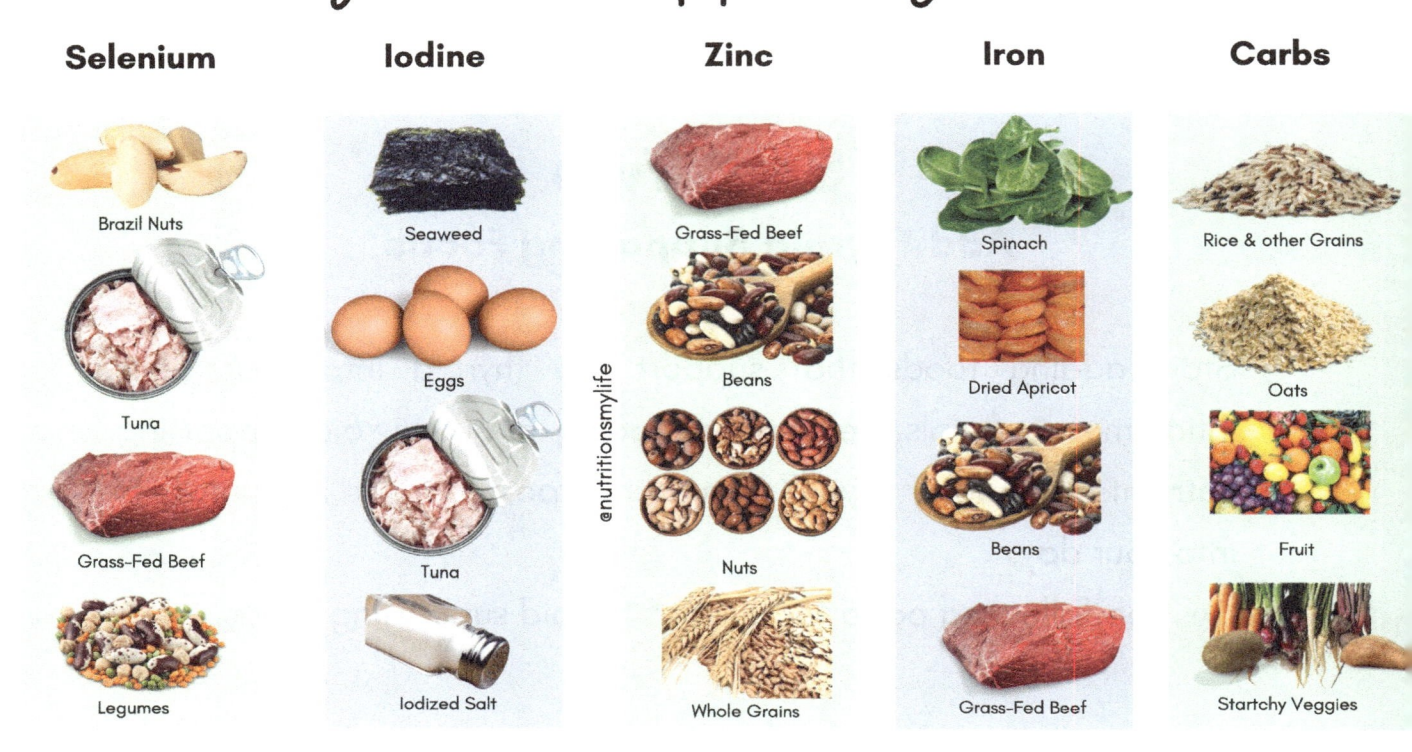

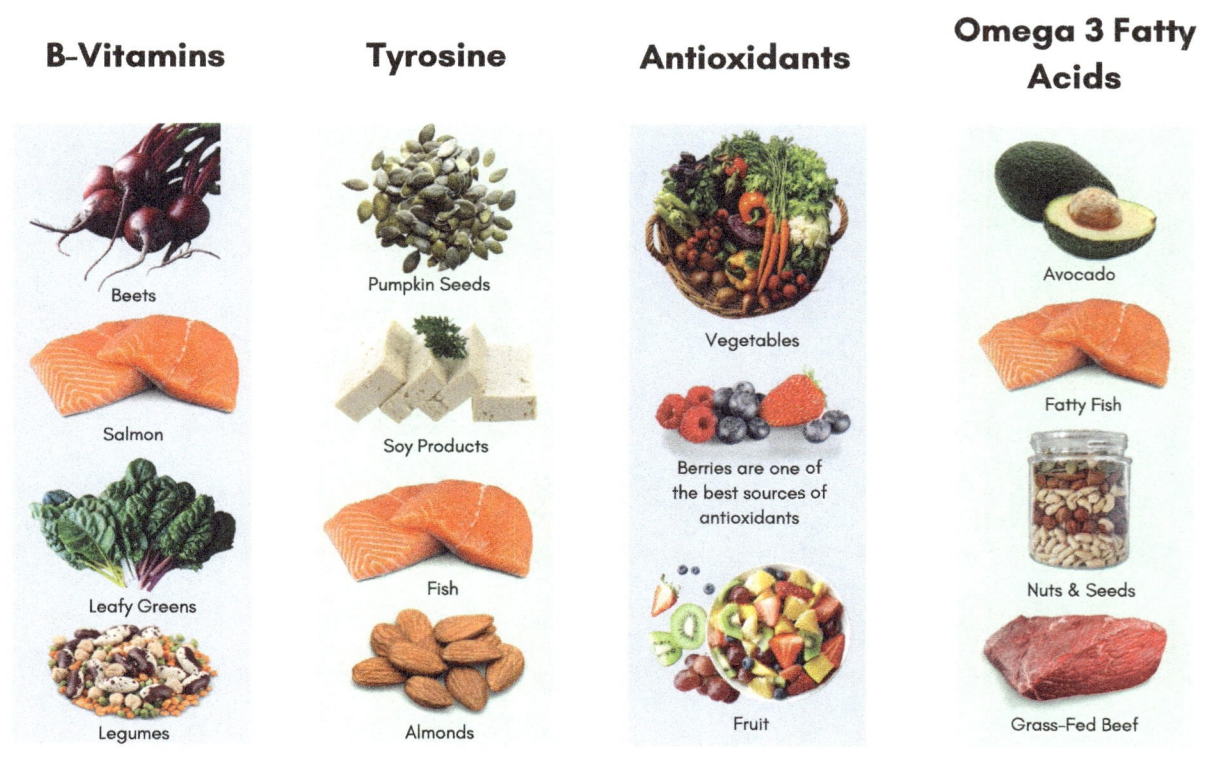

Selenium
- Brazil Nuts
- Tuna
- Grass-Fed Beef
- Legumes

Iodine
- Seaweed
- Eggs
- Tuna
- Iodized Salt

Zinc
- Grass-Fed Beef
- Beans
- Nuts
- Whole Grains

Iron
- Spinach
- Dried Apricot
- Beans
- Grass-Fed Beef

Carbs
- Rice & other Grains
- Oats
- Fruit
- Startchy Veggies

B-Vitamins
- Beets
- Salmon
- Leafy Greens
- Legumes

Tyrosine
- Pumpkin Seeds
- Soy Products
- Fish
- Almonds

Antioxidants
- Vegetables
- Berries are one of the best sources of antioxidants
- Fruit

Omega 3 Fatty Acids
- Avocado
- Fatty Fish
- Nuts & Seeds
- Grass-Fed Beef

How to eat for your thyroid

Step Three
Ensure Your Body is in the Rest & Digest Nervous System.

- If your body isn't in a calm state, you might just have expensive poop! What I mean is that you may not be absorbing or utilizing your nutrition properly. The body will not improve if it's stuck in the "fight or flight" response. One thing that can be easily overlooked is your stress level.
- Over the years I have seen a few common themes with the thyroid population:
    - Sweeping problems under the rug and not properly processing stress. This goes along with the following theme of, "I can do it all."
    - I can do it all and won't ask for help. This can include not asking a family member to watch your kid(s) for a moment to yourself. This can also be at work. Your boss might be asking you to do more, and mentally and physically you can't, but you say yes anyways.
    - You're very hard on yourself. You may be critical of your body, you may think you're not good enough, and decline compliments.

How to eat for your thyroid

Step Three

Ensure Your Body is in the Rest & Digest Nervous System.

- What these three common themes cause is internalized stress. If you're stuck in your fight or flight response, you're not going to heal. You might say, "I'm following an anti-inflammatory diet," but if your body is stuck in the wrong nervous system because of stress, you're not going to digest properly or recover. Stress is like someone turning the light switch off to the immune system.

Find what works for you to help stress less. If you keep going while under a large amount of stress, you're just going to have expensive poop because none of that nutrition is going to be working for you!

This is THE hardest part of all this, consistently putting yourself first and taking the time you need to get out of freak-out mode and into rest and digest! I find that most people who do go back into old, unhealthy habits do it because of stress (i.e. a move, a death in the family, etc.). Something stressful happens that sets them back.

How to eat for your thyroid

Step Three

Ensure body is in the Rest & Digest nervous system.

Case Study: A digestive health client improved her gut health to the point that she wasn't bloated, was pooping normal, and was successful with her weight loss goal. Three months after we stopped working together, she messaged me to say she had a lot of stress at work and started noticing some of her old symptoms again. She was able to recognize what was going on and got back on track fast using her stress reducing and digestive tools. She's now expecting her first child because her body is no longer stuck in her fight or flight nervous system anymore. The environment she created within her body was healthy enough to support another human being!

Pretty cool what the body is capable of when it's not stressed.

It's okay to: take breaks, ask for help, talk about what's bothering you, do more things that bring you joy, take deep belly breathes when you feel stressed, ground yourself, walk in nature, laugh so hard your cheeks hurt from smiling, see a therapist (I do!), etc. You're worth it!

Healthy Thyroid Meals Non-Negotiables

Per Meal

*The plate method helps reduce inflammation by promoting more antioxidants, balanced meals, and healthy fats.

- _ 3 colors on the plate
- _ a healthy fat option
- _ a source of complex carbs
- _ a quality protein source
- _ controlled portion sizes

Thyroid

*Choose at least one food from each thyroid supporting nutrient. Find food options for each nutrient 4 pages ago.

- _ Selenium
- _ Iodine
- _ Tyrosine
- _ Zinc
- _ B Vitamins
- _ Iron
- _ Carbs
- _ Antioxidants
- _ Omega 3 Fatty Acids

Chapter Ten

Supplements

Thyroid Supporting Supplements

> Please see your doctor and/or registered dietitian before starting a supplement regimen. Just because a supplement says it's helpful, doesn't mean it's the best option for you. Remember supplements can interact with medications and even certain foods. Everyone is different. There may be other supplements not listed here that may be beneficial. Please discuss supplements with your health professional. Visit www.nutritionsmylife.com/products-i-trust to for quality ingredient supplements.

Ashwagandha is an adaptogenic herb that is most notably known for its help with stress however it has been shown to be beneficial for many reasons such as brain health and Alzheimer's Disease. Ashwagandha is also beneficial for thyroid health. In a study, findings revealed that the ashwagandha root extract stimulates thyroidal activity and also enhances the antiperoxidation of hepatic tissue. Ashwagandha may be beneficial in treating hypothyroidism. 600 mg was the dose is this study (50).

Vitamin D supplementation is necessary in almost every patient I have worked with. Vitamin D is a fat soluble vitamin. This means it needs a fat source for absorption. I take mine with fish oil or with a meal that has a fat source. Please get your vitamin D level checked as dose is based off your lab results. Dose recommendations should only be from your health professional. See chapter seven for more information on vitamin D.

Thyroid Supporting Supplements

Probiotics are necessary for so many people to help replenish their ecosystem within their digestive tract! It's important to get a variety of different strains of probiotics. If you find a probiotic supplement with only one probiotic strain in it, put it back on the shelf and look for more! Look for a probiotic with multiple different strains of bacteria. Our digestive tract loves diversity.

Many of my clients that are in need of a lot of digestive repair benefit more from a spore-based probiotic, as they are not derived from dairy and tend to make it intact into the large intestine for optimal benefits.

When taking probiotics, please ensure adequate water intake in addition to fiber. If you don't have enough water throughout the day, you might not poop as often. Constipation is no fun. If water is difficult for you to remember to drink, get a big cup with a lid and straw. Most people drink more water with a straw. Keep that cup in eyesight all day long. Water helps so much.

See my website for probiotic options and talk to your health professional for guidance.

Thyroid Supporting Supplements

Magnesium is an important mineral that has over 300 roles in the body! There are many foods that contain magnesium like green leafy vegetables, nuts, seeds, tuna, avocado, and brown rice. Even though magnesium is so abundant in foods, only 30% to 40% of the dietary magnesium consumed is typically absorbed by the body (48). Most thyroid warriors have a higher demand for magnesium.

- People who have constipation may benefit from the form Magnesium Citrate.

- People who are stressed or have anxiety may benefit from Magnesium Glycinate or Magnesium Threonate.

- People with fibromyalgia or rheumatoid arthritis may benefit from Magnesium Taurate.

Personally, for my body, I eat a diet high in magnesium, take Magnesium Glycinate daily and take an Epsom salt bath three times a week for even more magnesium!

Magnesium needs are specific to our individual health conditions or demands. The RDA for Magnesium is set at 310-420 mg depending on age and sex.

Thyroid Supporting Supplements

Iron supplementation may be beneficial for some thyroid warriors if anemic. Poor gut health, taking proton pump inhibitors for heartburn, being vegetarian, or vegan all increase your risk of needing to take an iron supplement. Cooking in a cast iron skillet or even boiling an iron fish for increased iron intake may be beneficial.

Medicinal Mushrooms are also rich in selenium, a key antioxidant mineral for thyroid function too. I take Chaga for it's immune health qualities, antioxidants, and gut health benefits. Lion's Mane is my go to for my mood, nervous system, and brain health. Reishi is for better sleep. I take Freshcap Mushrooms and have for years! Many of my clients like their Thrive 6 blend. I am an affiliate for them now, use code NICOLE10 at checkout - find the link on my website's "product I trust" page.

Chapter Eleven

Recipes

The following recipes use the anti-inflammatory foods foundation diet and add thyroid supporting foods. I'm not a fan of meal plans as they restrict you to only eat what's scheduled. I want you to think about simply incorporating the foods we have discussed in this book and find ways to bring them into your day.

For Example:
- Pizza: add vegetables on top and have a salad on the side with seeds.
- Spaghetti: add spinach, mushrooms, zucchini and milled flaxseed.
- Your family's favorite go to recipe: ask yourself, "What color is missing?" and start adding in more vegetables based on colors that are lacking from a recipe.

Now, I don't want you to JUST use the following recipes. That gets boring after a while. Try updating your go-to recipes, or adapt that one recipe from social media you wanted to try, or replicate a meal you had at a restaurant. Get creative and incorporate thyroid supporting food where you can.

Recipes

When recipe hunting on your own, here are a few questions to ask yourself:

- How can I amplify this meal with more color?
- Do I have a source of healthy fat?
- Does this meal have a source of complex carbohydrates?
- Is my protein serving equal to the palm of my hand? (or smaller)

Dietitian Pro Tips

- Turn some music on and have a dance party while cooking! I have heard many people say they don't like to cook. But, when they turn on their favorite songs it makes a world of difference. Don't underestimate music and how it can positively impact your health.
- Make it a fun experience! If you have kids, try the rainbow game. The rainbow game is when you have the kids decorate their pizza or nachos with the colors of the rainbow.
- Picky eaters like to be in control and if they're not exposed to a food, then it can be scary. Present a few recipes with a variety of vegetables or highlighting a certain one. Then have them help cook that meal.

Thyroid Supporting Recipes

Smoothies are a great way to get a lot of nutrition! Here's an example of how to incorporate the anti-inflammatory foods + thyroid supporting foods together! This smoothie can easily replace a meal or be taken as a snack.

Berry Spice Smoothie
Thyroid & Gut Friendly
@Nutritionsmylife

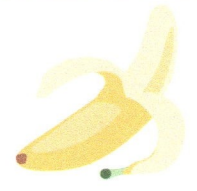

- 1/2 frozen banana
- 1/2 - 1 cup frozen blueberries
- 1 Tbsp nut butter
- probiotics (yogurt or open a supplement)
- handful of spinach
- 1/2 avocado
- 1 tsp cinnamon
- 1 Tbsp milled flaxseed
- 1/2 - 1 cooked beet or beet juice
- 1 cup non-dairy milk

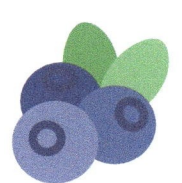

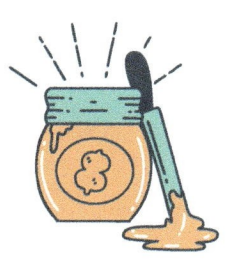

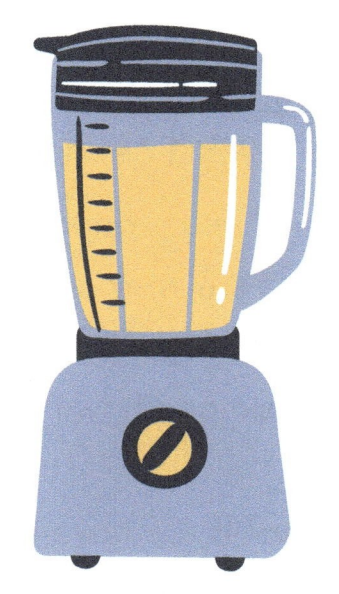

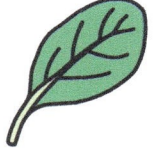

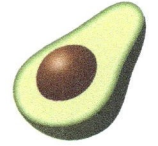

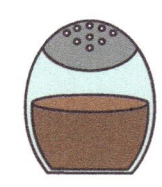

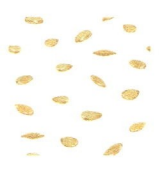

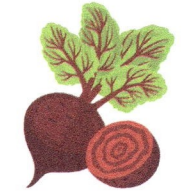

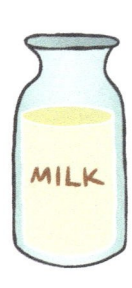

Food For Thought

What if you start looking at food for what it can do for you instead of how many calories or carbs it has?

Look at what this thyroid supporting smoothie provides:

<u>Banana:</u> For sweetness and provides you with potassium and magnesium.

<u>Blueberries:</u> Delicious in taste and provides you with antioxidants to help reduce damage to your cells, plus supports a healthy liver for that T4 to T3 conversion.

<u>Nut Butter (Cashew or Almond Butter preferred):</u> Provides you with protein, healthy fats for inflammation reduction, zinc, selenium, and copper for thyroid health.

<u>Probiotics:</u> To help digest the fiber in this smoothie and support healthy digestion.

<u>Spinach:</u> Loaded with iron for thyroid health, glutathione for liver support, and chlorophyll for cellular support.

<u>Avocado:</u> For healthy fats to help inflammation reduction and magnesium for stress reduction.

<u>Cinnamon:</u> For flavor and inflammation reduction.

<u>Milled Flaxseed:</u> For fiber, healthy fats, and heart health due to cholesterol reduction.

<u>Beets:</u> Provides complex carbs and for liver support as they contain high amounts of glutathione and are great energy boosting foods!

<u>Non-Dairy Milk or Water:</u> For liquid – add more or less based on preferred consistency.

Turmeric Latte

Ingredients

- 8oz warm/hot almond milk
- 1 Tbsp turmeric
- 2 tsp cinnamon
- 1 tsp ginger
- pinch black pepper
- 1 tsp local honey or maple syrup

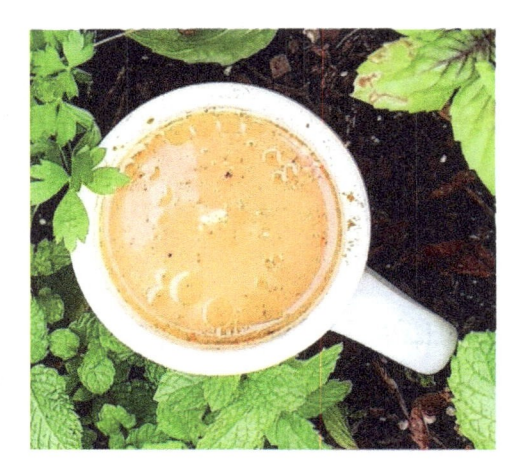

Directions

1. Heat up milk of choice to desired temperature.
2. Add spices and use frother to mix.
3. Add sweetness of choice and froth latte again.
4. Add any additional inflammation reduction tools, like medicinal mushrooms.

Dietitian Pro Tip:

Try swapping out your morning coffee for an inflammation reducing latte.

Turmeric Latte

Why a turmeric latte?

Curcumin is found in **Turmeric** and has been extensively studied. It downregulates MULTIPLE inflammatory pathways (52). Meaning it blocks inflammation from occurring.

In low doses, curcumin can regulate antibody response. Meaning turmeric is helpful for allergies, asthma, Alzheimer's disease, diabetes, and immune disorders.

I drink a turmeric latte every morning. I actually encourage most of my clients to start their day with this drink. I've been told that this drink has helped with energy and inflammation. I drink it as I have arthritis and can easily get migraines if I don't have a diet rich in anti-inflammatory foods. I add medicinal mushrooms to mine as well. Medicinal mushrooms are rich in antioxidants and also have anti-inflammatory properties.

There are many different kinds of medicinal mushrooms and before anyone asks, no, they're not psychedelic mushrooms. Some mushrooms like chaga are great for inflammation reduction and immune health (53). If you have anxiety, like me, reishi mushrooms may be beneficial. Reishi may help with calmness, relaxation, and more specifically, sleep (54).

Thyroid Breakfast Recipes

Blueberry Omega 3 Breakfast Bars

Base:
- 2 cups old fashioned oats
- 1 cup crushed walnuts
- 4 Tbsp honey or maple syrup
- 4 Tbsp milled flaxseed
- 1 Tbsp coconut oil
- 1 tsp kosher salt
- 2 tsp cinnamon
- 2 bananas
- 1 1/2 tsp vanilla extract
- 2 scoops organic vanilla protein powder or hydrolyzed collagen / collagen peptides

Topping:
- 1/2 cup old fashioned oats
- 1/4 cup walnuts
- 1/4 cup pumpkin seeds
- 1 cup fresh organic blueberries
- 1/4 cup of almond milk
- 1/4 tsp cinnamon

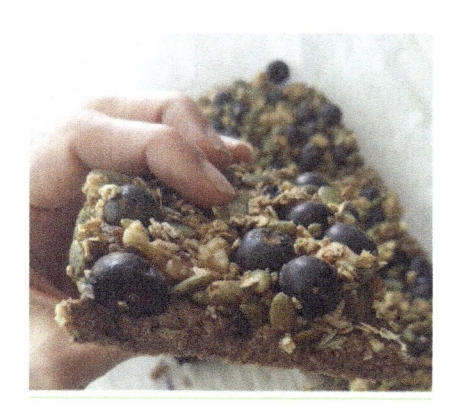

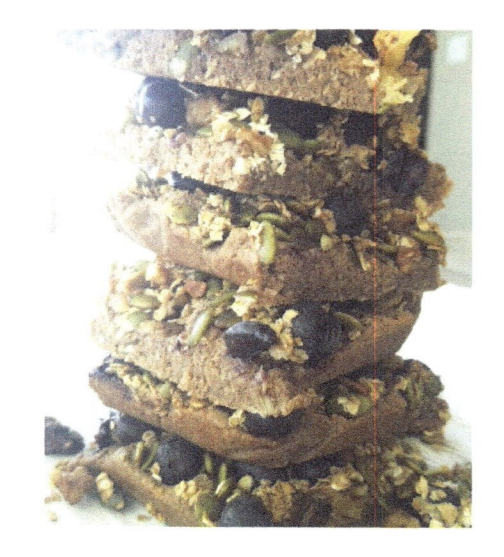

Thyroid Breakfast Recipes

Blueberry Omega 3 Breakfast Bars

Base Instructions:

1. Preheat the oven to 350°F.
2. Line 9x9-inch baking pan with parchment paper.
3. Add all ingredients into the food processor until completely combined and wet. This may take several minutes.
4. Pour into the prepared pan and smooth out with a spatula until evenly spread.
5. Bake for 8 - 10 minutes. Remove from the oven and follow the topping's instructions.

Topping Instructions:

1. Place ingredients in medium bowl and stir to combine.
2. Remove pan from oven, and spread the topping evenly.
3. Press down into base.
4. Bake for an additional 15 minutes.
5. Cut into 6 squares & store in an airtight container for up to a week in the fridge.

Serving options:
- Eat 1 square + fruit & hard boiled egg for breakfast
- 2 squares on the go
- 1 square + 1/2 cup yogurt with fruit
- 1 square as a snack

Crumbs
You will inevitably have crumbs from the toppings falling off. SAVE THEM! Use the crumbs as toppings to oatmeal or yogurt!!

Easy Breakfast Options

Sweet Potato Taco

Ingredients

- Sweet potato
- Cherry tomatoes
- Avocado & salsa
- Cilantro & green onion
- Protein source: fried egg and/or black beans

Directions

1. Poke holes in potato, wrap in wet paper towel, and cook in microwave for 7 – 9 minutes.
2. While the sweet potato is cooking, chop up the remainder of the ingredients, and heat up the beans or cook an egg.
3. Place ingredients in cooked sweet potato and there's your taco. Yum!

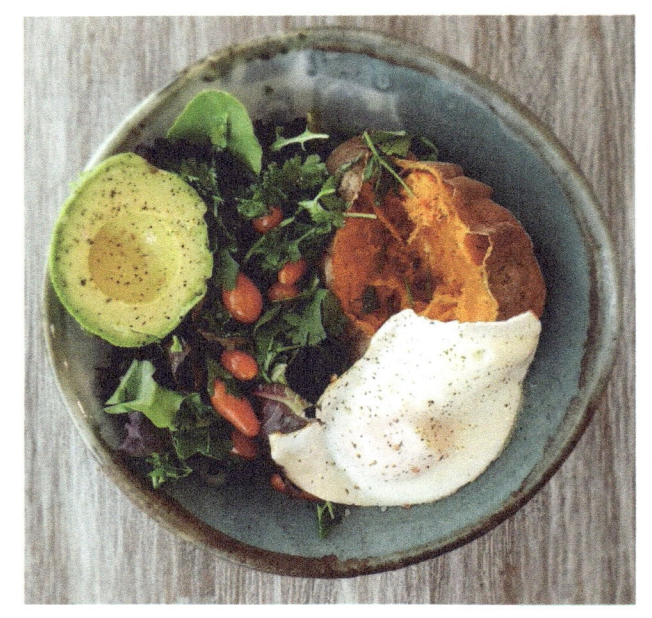

Easy Breakfast Options

Yogurt or Oatmeal Parfait

- Dairy free or grass – fed Greek yogurt

OR

- Oatmeal parfait: your base will be steel cut oats + enough dairy free milk to cover oats.
- 1 tsp – 1 Tbsp of milled flaxseed
- 1 tsp local honey
- 1/4 cup – 1/2 cup walnuts
- 1/2 cup berries

*For oatmeal, it needs more protein: add cashew butter or your favorite protein powder.

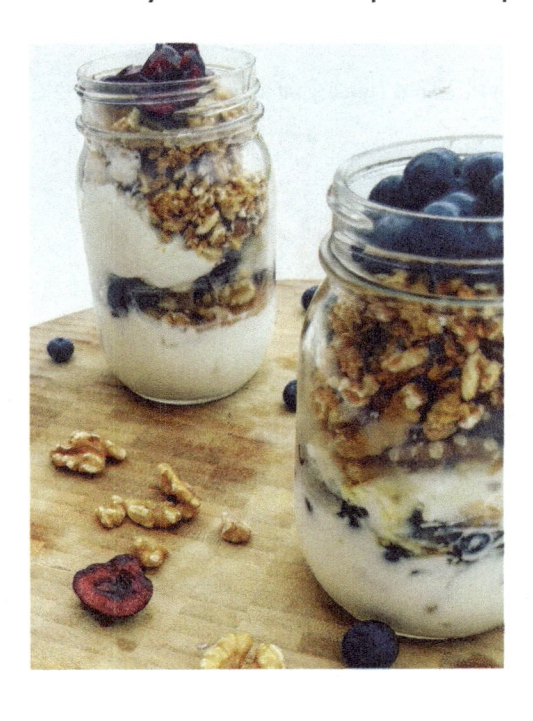

Thyroid Snack Options

Being hungry enough in between meals for a snack is always a great sign your metabolism is working! Sometimes, though, you may not be hungry enough for a meal and only have room for a snack. No matter the reason behind a snack, it's a good idea to make sure you're pairing your snacks properly. Carbs should always be paired with a protein and/or fat source.

See below and the next few pages for examples.

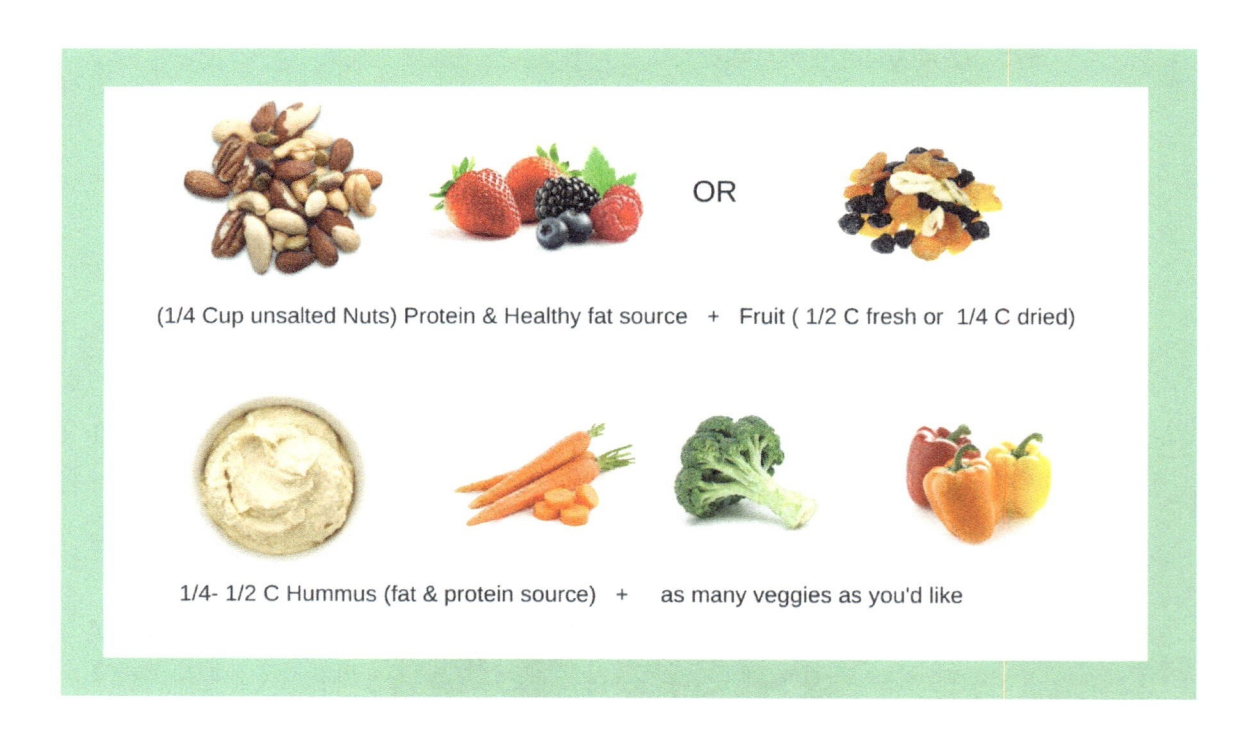

(1/4 Cup unsalted Nuts) Protein & Healthy fat source   +   Fruit (1/2 C fresh or 1/4 C dried)   OR

1/4- 1/2 C Hummus (fat & protein source)   +   as many veggies as you'd like

Thyroid Snack Options

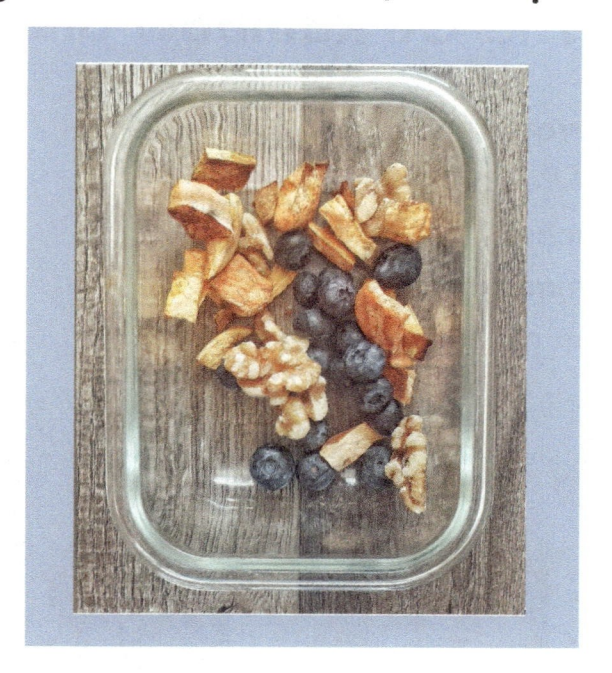

Walnuts + Blueberries + Cinnamon sweet potato bites

1. Cut sweet potato into bite size chunks. You can choose to add a drizzle of avocado oil to the sweet potatoes to help with cinnamon sticking more but I find that it works well without.
2. Sprinkle with cinnamon
3. Roast sweet potatoes at 400° F in the oven for 15 – 20 mins.
4. Let cool and then mix with blueberries and walnuts for a delicious snack.

Thyroid Snack Options

On-The-Go Rainbow Snacks

- Carrots
- Bell Peppers
- Broccoli
- Hummus made from olive oil
- Nuts
- Fruit
- Cheese

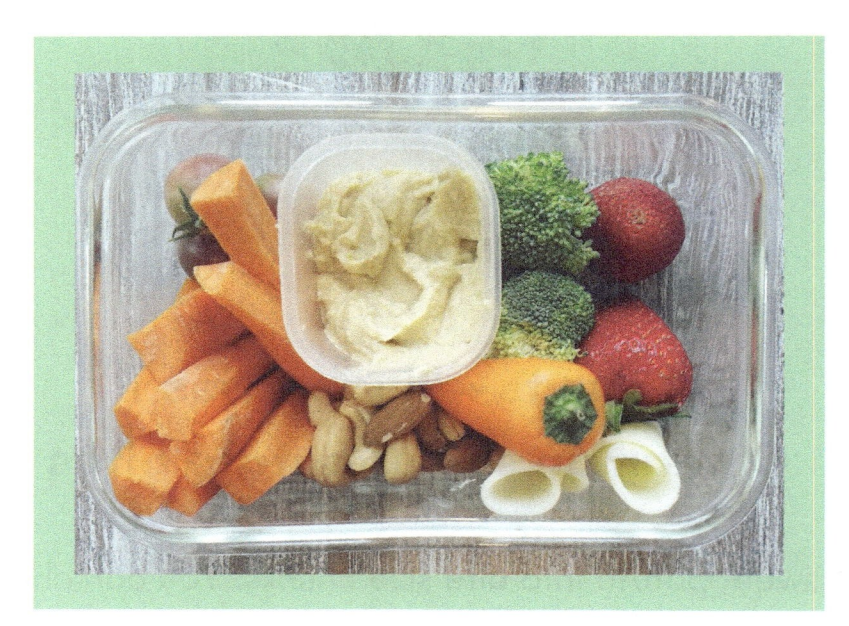

Dietitian Pro Tips:

- Broccoli and other cruciferous vegetables need to be cooked for thyroid warriors most of the time.
- Dairy can promote inflammation, limit to a few times a week.
- This can easily be a lunch if larger portions are included.
- Swap out ingredients as you like however consider how colorful this is and the fact it's following the plate method.

Thyroid Snack Options

Sweet and Savory Toast

- Avocado whole wheat or gluten-free toast with salt, red pepper flakes (avoid if you have digestive issues) and top with pumpkin seeds.

- Cashew or almond butter toast with blueberries, cinnamon, and a drizzle of local honey

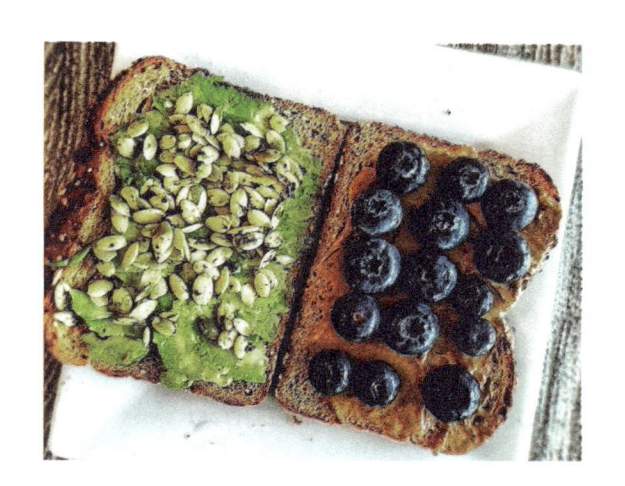

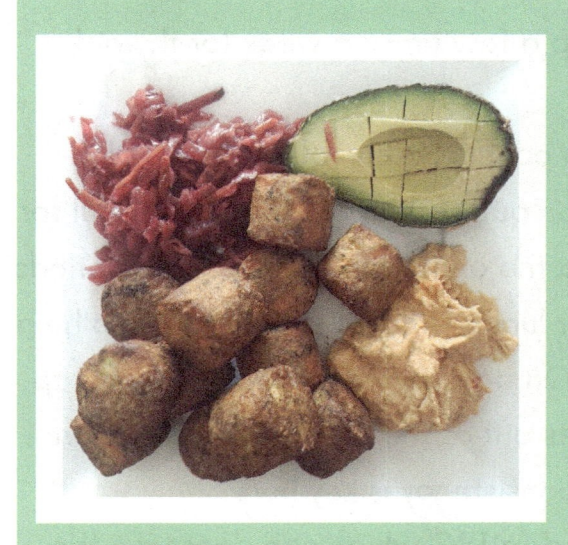

Veggie Bites With Fermented Beets

- Veggie Bites (Costco)
- Hummus (bonus if you can find it made with olive oil!
- Fermented Beets (for liver support)
- 1/2 Avocado

Veggie & Hummus Wrap

Ingredients

- 1 flavored wrap or tortilla, I used spinach
- 1/3 cup hummus
- Bell peppers sliced lengthwise
- Handful of fresh spinach
- 1 sliced tomato
- 1/4 of an avocado sliced
- Fresh broccoli sprouts
- Fresh microgreens
- Basil leaves, if desired

Directions

1. Spread the hummus on the bottom 1/3 of the wrap, about 1/2 inch from the bottom edge but spreading out the side edges.
2. Layer the bell peppers, spinach, tomato slices, avocado slices, broccoli sprouts, microgreens and basil.
3. Fold the wrap tightly, as you would a burrito, tucking in all of the veggies with the first roll then rolling firmly to the end.
4. Eat with a side of roasted sea weed

Dietitian Pro Tips

- Turn this wrap into a **tuna** wrap a few times a week for thyroid health!
- Broccoli sprouts contain a high concentration of DIM (55). DIM assists with detoxifying estrogen out of the body. This is helpful for people with high estrogen (aka the ones with really painful periods).
- Adding broccoli sprouts to your lunch wraps is an easy way to help with your hormone balancing. On days you're not eating the wrap, simply grab a handful of sprouts out of the fridge and munch on them! Like with anything else, consistency is key here.
- High levels of estrogen can bind to TBG which can decrease the amount of T3 available for you, making you feel even more tired & run down!

Cheeseburger & Sweet Potato Fries

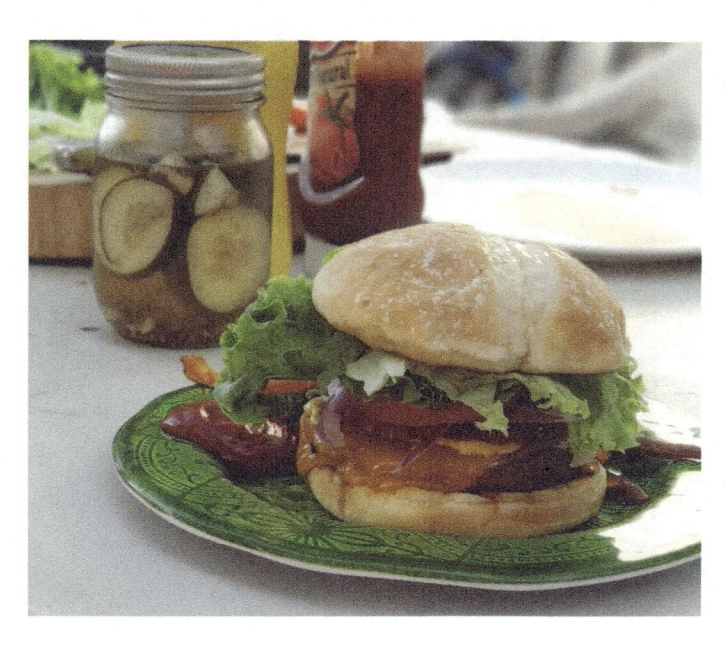

- Black bean burger (I get mine from Costco)

OR

- Grass-fed beef patties
- Cheddar or provolone cheese (1 slice)
- Tomato & lettuce
- Onions thinly sliced
- Pickles
- Potato or whole wheat bun
- Sweet potato, cut into fries
- Avocado oil

This burger can be made with grass-fed beef or with your favorite veggie burger. Be aware of the ingredients in the veggies burger, avoid processed soy. Either grill the burger up outside or cook inside on medium-high heat. I like cheese but like to minimize the amount I eat, so throughout this guide you'll see cheese included only occasionally.

Serve with a side of homemade fries. Cut the potato thin lengthwise and place on a sheet pan. Drizzle with avocado oil and a pinch of salt (sometimes I'll add Cajun seasoning instead of salt) and roast at 425°F for about 20 minutes.

Rainbow Pizza

Naan Bread Pizza

- Whole wheat naan bread or GF if needed
- Spaghetti sauce (save remainder of jar for spaghetti)
- Any veggies you like
- Mozzarella cheese (bonus points if you can find grass-fed cheese)
- Uncured pepperoni
- Fresh basil and oregano

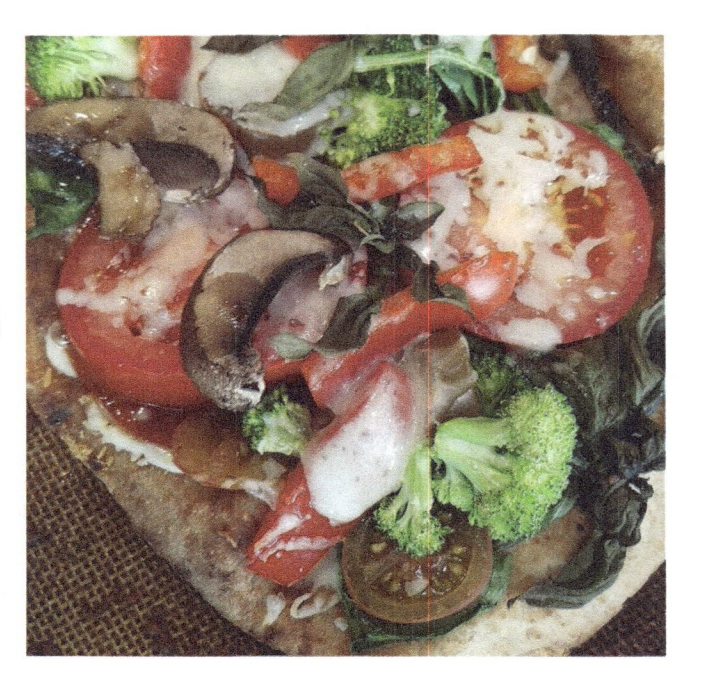

Serving: 1 naan bread pizza per person

Directions

1. Preheat the oven to 425°F
2. Top naan bread with spaghetti sauce.
3. Add any vegetables you'd like, we like to aim for the rainbow!
4. Then add fresh basil and very little cheese on top!
5. Bake for 10-15 minutes (keep an eye on it!).
6. Once out of the oven, drizzle with olive oil and garlic.
7. Then add even more oregano and basil.

This is a fun family meal; it's a great way to get the kids to choose their vegetables for their own pizza!

Thyroid Friendly Recipes

Sheet Pan Salmon

- Wild caught salmon
- Sweet potato, cubed
- Zucchini, cut in discs
- Baby portobello mushrooms, cleaned & cut in half
- Avocado oil
- Grass-fed butter
- Garlic, chopped
- Cinnamon
- Salt & pepper to taste

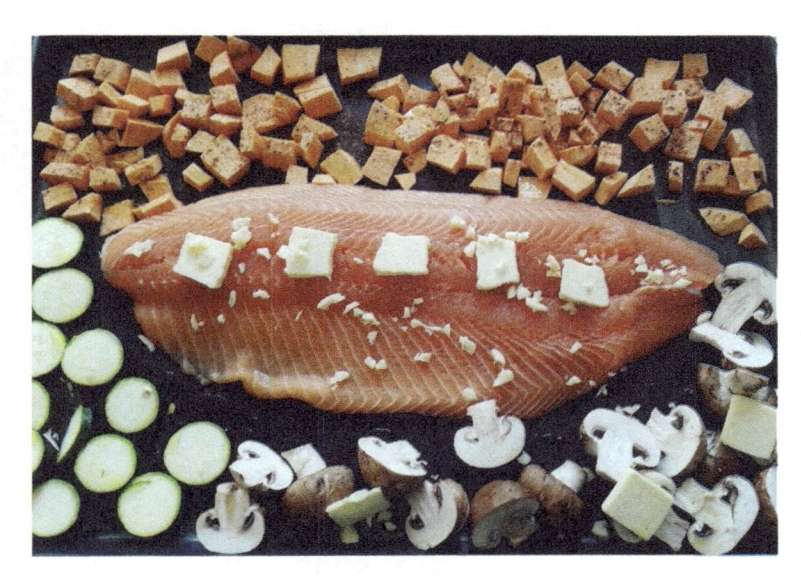

Directions:

1. Preheat Oven to 425°F
2. Line sheet pan and ingredients to look like the picture.
3. Put avocado oil & cinnamon on the sweet potatoes.
4. Add more avocado oil and garlic on the other veggies.
5. Add butter and garlic to salmon
6. Cook for 15 minutes (if your salmon is small in size, you may want to cook the veggies for 10 minutes by themselves and then add the salmon for the remainder of time)

Thyroid Friendly Recipes

Sheet Pan Steak and Veggies

- 2 lbs baby red potatoes
- 1 head of broccoli, largely chopped
- 2 Tbsp avocado oil
- 1 - 2 Tbsp garlic powder
- 1 tsp dried thyme
- Kosher salt and freshly ground black pepper, to taste
- 1 lb (1 inch thick) top sirloin steak, patted dry

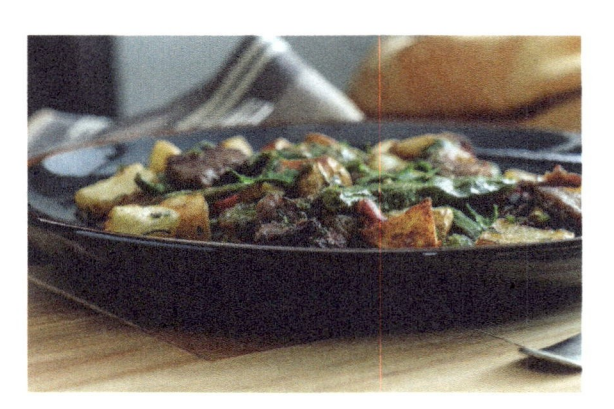

Directions

1. Preheat the oven to broil and grease the sheet pan.
2. In a large pot, boil potatoes for 12 - 15 minutes; drain well.
3. Put potatoes and broccoli on a sheet pan . Add avocado oil, garlic and thyme. Season with salt and pepper, to taste. Gently toss to combine.
4. Season steaks with salt and pepper, to taste. Add to a sheet pan in a single layer. Place into oven and broil until the steak is browned and charred at the edges (about 4 - 5 minutes per side for medium-rare, longer for well-done).
5. Serve immediately with optional garlic butter

Spaghetti

Ingredients

- 1 pound grass-fed ground beef
- 1 onion, chopped
- 4 cloves garlic, minced
- 1 large zucchini, diced
- Handful chopped broccoli
- 2 cups baby portobello mushrooms, cut in fourths
- 1 (28 ounce) can diced tomatoes
- 1 jar organic spaghetti sauce
- 1 (6 ounce) can tomato paste
- 3 Tbsp milled flaxseed
- 2 tsp dried oregano
- 2 tsp dried basil
- 1 tsp salt
- ½ tsp black pepper

Directions

1. Combine ground beef, onion, and garlic in a large saucepan. Cook on medium heat and stir until meat is brown and vegetables are tender. Drain grease.
2. Stir zucchini, mushrooms, broccoli, diced tomatoes, tomato sauce, and tomato paste into the pan. Season with oregano, basil, salt, and pepper. Simmer spaghetti sauce for 1 hour, stirring occasionally.
3. Add the flaxseed. Stir again and serve over noodles.
4. Cook noodles per package directions. Whole wheat noodles, durum or semolina wheat, gluten free, lentil or chickpea pasta are all good options.

Tofu Pad Thai

Ingredients

- 1 package firm tofu
- 8 oz wide rice noodles
- 1 red bell pepper, julienne style
- 3 green onions
- 1 large carrot, thinly sliced
- 4 garlic cloves, minced
- 2 eggs beaten
- ½ cup ground peanuts
- ½ c cilantro leaves, chopped
- ½ lime juiced

Sauce

- ¼ cup local honey
- 2 Tbsp low sodium soy sauce
- 2 Tbsp lime juice
- 2 Tbsp rice wine vinegar
- 2 Tbsp peanut butter
- ½ tsp dried basil (fresh is best if you have some!)
- ½ tsp coriander powder
- ½ tsp ground ginger
- ¼ tsp pepper

*Add your own spice of preference. Chili paste, red pepper flakes, special sauce etc. Most of my recipes are kid friendly.

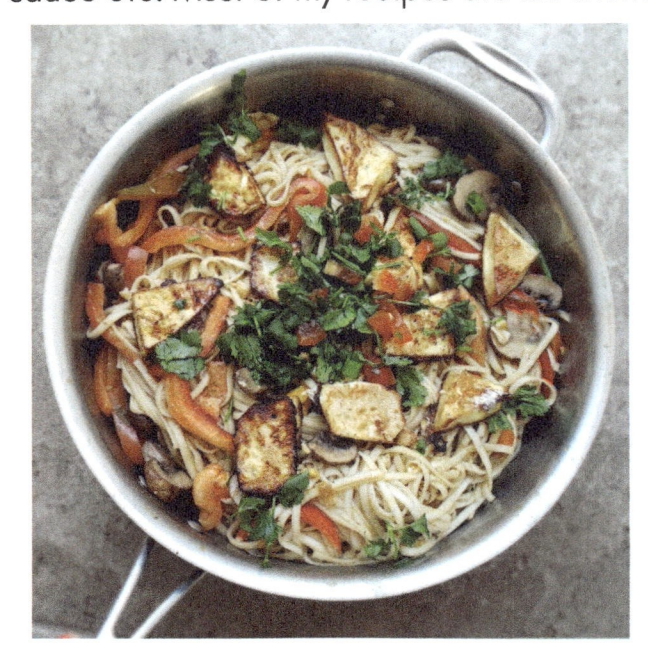

Tofu Pad Thai
Directions

1. Preheat the oven to 400° F and drain the tofu.
2. Dry tofu off with towels. Try to get it as dry as you can but be careful not to push too hard or you'll burst it open (don't ask me how I know this ;))
3. Once tofu is dried, cut it in half so it will cook faster.
4. Place onto a sheet pan. Drizzle with soy sauce and honey. How much? ... a drizzle (up to your taste). Then place in the oven 10 – 15 minutes before they need to be flipped.
5. Make your sauce by going down the ingredient list. Plop them all in a bowl and mix them together. The honey should dissolve fairly fast with all that acidity in there!
6. Thinly chop up your vegetables.
7. Turn the sauté pan on medium to medium high heat. Add in mushrooms first and keep an eye on them. Around this time you'll need to flip the tofu if you haven't already done so – (use your nose a little. It will start to burn, so you'll want to catch it right before that. I promise if you use your sense of smell you'll be able to figure out the right timing).
8. Boil a large pot of water for your noodles and cook al dente. You'll want to keep an eye on them. I stir them occasionally in between moving my mushrooms around.
9. Next, add your green onions and garlic. Let them mix with the mushrooms for a bit and then add your red bell peppers in.
10. Make a hole in the middle of the veggies in the sauté pan and crack 2 eggs into the middle. Reduce heat to low and scramble eggs. Then mix with the veggies.
11. Add in your noodles and sauce to the pan. Increase your heat a little and toss until evenly combined.
12. Add your toppings: Tofu, cilantro, green onions, peanuts, and lime.

Sheet Pan Meal Cheat Sheet

Preheat oven to 425°F. You'll need a sheet pan, sheet pan liner (parchment paper or silicone mat), and music for dancing.

Food Mood — combine in bowl & sprinkle over meal before roasting

Indian: 1 Tbsp turmeric, 2 tsp ground ginger, 1 tsp cinnamon

Italian: 2 Tbsp olive oil or avocado oil, zest of 1 lemon, 3 minced garlic cloves, chopped parsley and oregano.

Mexican: 2 tsp cumin, 3 garlic cloves minced *add tsp paprika or cilantro, lime juice optional* flavor heat: jalapenos

Thai: ginger, cilantro, lime

Protein — serving size is individualized based on palm of hand

Salmon, large shrimp
Grass-fed beef (ribeye, meatballs)
Air chilled chicken breast (antibiotic free)

Black beans, garbanzo beans, red beans, edamame, lentils (beans & lentils cooked per package directions and not on sheet pan)

Whole Grain — Serving size Adult: 1/2 cup Child: 1/3 cup

Barley, brown rice, oats, quinoa, freekeh, whole wheat tortillas
Cook per package directions & not on sheet pan.

Vegetables: Choose 3 colors/meal — Serving size 1 cup minimum

Have veggies cubed and oiled + food mood seasoned, before adding to sheet pan

Reds: bell peppers, beets, onions, potatoes, radishes, radicchio, tomato
Orange: Bell peppers, carrots, squash (acorn, butternut, winter), sweet potatoes
Yellow: Bell pepper, corn on the cob, Summer Squash
Green: Asparagus, bell peppers, broccoli, bok choy, brussel sprouts, cabbage, green beans, okra, and zucchini
Blue/purple/black: Cabbage, carrots, cauliflower, eggplant, potatoes
White/tan/brown: Cauliflower, mushrooms, onions, shallots

Toppings — Serving size per person 1 Tbsp or less

Cranberries, raisins (black or golden), cherries, goji berries, local honey, lemon & lime juice

Nuts and Seeds — Nuts: 1/4 cup per person Seeds: 1 Tbsp per person

Nuts: Walnuts, pistachios, pecans, cashews
Seeds: Milled flax seed, chia seeds, sunflower seeds, sprouted pumpkin seeds

Healthy Fats — serving size 1-2 Tbsp

Avocado, greek yogurt, nuts/seed, hummus, grass-fed butter, olive oil, avocado oil, olives

Most meals take 30 mins to roast but may be done in 20 mins depending on thickness. Make sure protein temp is 165°F minimum before eating. Sheet Pan Meals can turn into quinoa bowls, tacos, stir fries etc., be creative.

Nutrition's My Life (c) all rights reserved

Sheet Pan Veggie Bowls

The sheet pan "recipes" you see on the next page are my go to for many nights out of the week because they're fast and easy. I always make too much, so I can have leftover for lunches! I call these my VEGGIE BOWLS. Think layers! Start with your grains, whole wheat pastas, or lentil/bean pastas (~1/2 cup serving). Then layer with veggies (aim for 2-3 colors), beans, and/or animal protein source (tuna, salmon, grass-fed beef), fresh herb or green onion, plus a sauce and a source of healthy fat. Many times, I'll add raw veggies for extra crunch. If you're having digestive issues stick with roasted veggies.

Swap out different veggies each time you make these bowls. Add seeds for crunch, magnesium, zinc, and healthy fats . Use the cheat sheet on the previous page to find your favorite combinations.
As you'll find, there are many different variations to try!!
Pro Tip: Play music while cooking and start enjoying the process!

Veggie Bowl Directions

1. Cook desired amount of brown or wild rice, quinoa or lentil/whole wheat pasta (GF if applicable). Serving size cooked is ~1/4 - 1/2 cup for adults depending on activity level and if weight loss is desired. Amount of rice you'll cook up will be based on how many times you're going to have leftovers for the week.
2. Preheat the oven to 400° F
3. Add cut up veggies to the lined sheet pan, drizzle with avocado oil, garlic powder or desired seasonings.
4. Roast veggies for about 20 minutes and meats/seafood until desired internal temperature is met. (When I cook with seafood, I typically wait until the veggies are halfway done cooking and then add the seafood so it doesn't overcook.)
5. Combine your grains with veggies, protein source, fat, and always aim to top with fresh herbs and onion, if your digestion can tolerate it.

Veggie Bowls

Tuna Veg N Beans Bowl

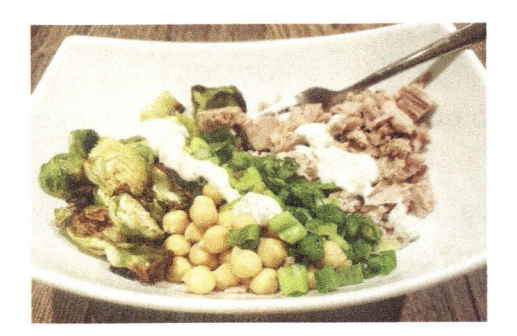

- Skip jack tuna
- Cooked brown rice
- Brussels sprouts
- Garbanzo beans
- Green onion, chopped
- Homemade ranch dressing or hummus
- Salt and pepper to taste

Mexican Veggie Bowl

- Black beans
- Cooked brown rice or quinoa
- Sweet potatoes roasted, cubed
- Bell peppers, roasted
- Tomatoes, diced
- Corn, cooked or canned
- Red onions, diced
- Avocado, diced
- Cilantro and green onion, chopped
- Homemade ranch dressing mixed with salsa

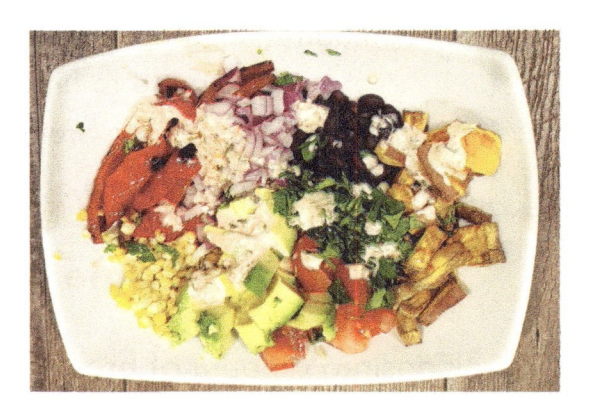

Cajun Shrimp Veggie Bowl

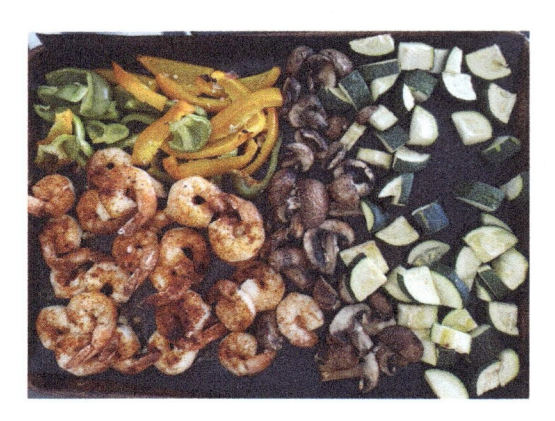

- No shell deveined shrimp
- Bell peppers, julienne cut
- Mushrooms, cleaned & cut in half
- Zucchinis, cut same size as shrooms
- Cooked brown rice or quinoa
- Tony Chachere's Creole Seasoning, or your favorite go to Cajun spices.
- Parsley and chopped celery as garnish

Chapter Twelve

Healthy Thyroid Non-Negotiables Check List

Do the best you can with what you have!

Don't try to do everything in this book at once! I think a lot of times people get overwhelmed after reading through educational information and then trying to implement EVERYTHING at once. It ends in failure.

Start where you feel you need the most help.

Do you need gut health help? Maybe you start incorporating more probiotic rich foods (fermented foods), cook your vegetables, and increase your water.

Are you tired? Maybe you start incorporating more anti-inflammatory foods first and then tackle stress/anxiety, so you can sleep better.

As much as I'd like to say, do this step first and this next... it's really not that simple as we're all different. We all have different needs. Start with focusing on two to three things a week. This could be just starting to eat breakfast, adding in more color into your plate, or taking a probiotic.

Start small, get confident in the new habit, and then continue to add more into your day.

Healthy Thyroid Non-Negotiables Check List

Nutrition

- Plate Method Used for portion sizes at meals
- Included Anti-Inflammatory Foods
- Thyroid Supporting Foods
    - Hypothyroidism / Hashimoto's Disease
        - Include thyroid supporting nutrients listed in chapter nine
    - Hyperthyroidism / Graves Disease
        - Minimal Tyrosine Foods
        - Minimal Iodine Rich Foods

Gut Health

- Water
- Probiotics
- Fiber
- Less Stress
- Movement
- Pooping is easy and come out like a snake

Lifestyle Factors

- Deep Sleep is consistently achieved
- Stress Reduction
- Decrease of Endocrine Disruptors
- Exercise is appropriate to health/stress of body

Example of my healthy thyroid day

I'm giving you an insight into my M-F life in hopes you'll be able to see how these tools may fit into your life easier than you think!!

Morning Routine

Habits	Time	Food
• Gratitude upon waking (I think about how grateful for the bed, the fan, the sun shining through the window, my husband & kids etc) • Supplements + water • Read by open window & open door for sunlight OR workout in garage w/husband OR go for 1-2hr hike after I drop the kids off at school • Help kids get ready for school • Work • Take breaks in between clients or projects (breaks include 5-10 minutes of stretching or walking outside/working in my garden to help with stress of the day)	5:45 am 6:00 am 6:30 am 7:30 am	• water • turmeric latte • brazil nuts • If I go on a hike, will eat a banana or small bowl of oatmeal • Breakfast many mornings is a sweet potato taco, leftovers from the night before, or sweet and savory toast with fruit on the side.

Day Routine

Habits	Time	Food

• Stress Reduction Tools:
  ◦ Take breaks in between clients or projects (breaks include 5-10 minutes of stretching or walking outside/working in my garden)
  ◦ If needed; boxed breathing or grounding to help decrease anxiety
• Music playing in the background while I work.
• Take breaks to play with kids or do housework.
	10:30 am
	
	1:30 pm
	
	3:30 pm
	
	4:30 pm
		• Snack: walnuts with an orange or salsa with avocado and chips
		
		• Lunch: Leftover dinner or will make tuna if I don't have any leftovers. Sometimes if the leftovers aren't enough volume or contains enough vegetables, I might cook a vegetable in the air fryer while I'm working to add to lunch. Top my meals a lot of times with fermented beets.
		
		• Snack: pumpkin seeds and a piece of fruit

Evening Routine

Habits	Time	Food

• Stretch! After a long day of working at my desk, I always end my work day with stretching. I also prioritize being outside to de-stress.
• Turn on music to enjoy the process of cooking more.
• Write at least one thing down on my "It Matter's Board". This is my way of focusing on the positives and what is going well for me.
• Blue light canceling glasses to block any light illuminating from my phone, tv, or computer. This will help me sleep better.
• Read or draw after I put the kids to sleep.
	5:45 pm
	
	6:00 pm
	
	7:00 pm
	
	8:30 pm
	
	9:00 pm
		• Start chopping up vegetables and preheat the oven for a sheet pan meal dinner.
		  ◦ In pot on stove: brown rice
		  ◦ Chop and place on sheet pan: broccoli, mushrooms, sugar snap peas, tomato, carrots
		  ◦ Add salmon with herb butter 10 minutes after veggies started cooking at 400°F
		  ◦ Eat Dinner
		• Dessert: frozen cherries, chocolate chips, and a few walnuts

My healthy thyroid day

Fill in this blank day with habits and foods that you feel may benefit you from this Healthy Thyroid Guide.

Morning Routine

Habits   Food

Day Routine

Habits   Food

Evening Routine

Habits   Food

My healthy thyroid day

Fill in this blank day with habits and foods that you feel may benefit you from this Healthy Thyroid Guide.

Morning Routine

Habits								Food

Day Routine

Habits								Food

Evening Routine

Habits								Food

My healthy thyroid day

Fill in this blank day with habits and foods that you feel may benefit you from this Healthy Thyroid Guide.

Morning Routine

Habits   Food

Day Routine

Habits   Food

Evening Routine

Habits   Food

Healthy Thyroid Food Diary

Listen to your gut!

Food diary time! When you're learning to listen to your body, take note of how food and mood affects your body. What were you doing before and during eating? How were you feeling before, during, and after eating? How did the food make you feel?

Part of keeping a food diary is to help tune into your digestion, but another part is to identify your body cues, like more energy or bloating.

HUNGER is a cue. Not something we ignore or push aside yet that is something I hear so frequently in my practice. So it gets ignored and then "HOLY COW I'M STARVING" and then poor food choices happen. Which triggers you to feel guilty about what happened. Sound about right?

This is why being mindful is so important. Hunger is a GOOD thing. It's a sign that your metabolism is working and –guess what?– once your metabolism is working at a better rate for you– you'll be hungrier! This is why listening to how foods respond inside your body is crucial!

Healthy Thyroid Food Diary

Here are some questions to ask yourself:

1. How does that food make me feel?
2. Did that meal give me energy?
3. Did that meal make me feel sluggish?
4. Am I full?
5. What about my meal made me hungry shortly after I was done eating?
6. How was I FEELING before the meal *(remember being stressed, angry, depressed, etc. can shunt blood away from your digestive tract making foods harder to digest/tolerate.)*

Use the provided Food and Feel Journal pages to help tune into how food responds to your body.

Food & Feel Journal

	MEAL I ATE	MY MOOD	HOW IT MADE ME FEEL	OTHER THINGS I NOTICED
BREAKFAST				
LUNCH				
SNACK				
DINNER				

Food & Feel Journal

	MEAL I ATE	MY MOOD	HOW IT MADE ME FEEL	OTHER THINGS I NOTICED
BREAKFAST				
LUNCH				
SNACK				
DINNER				

Food & Feel Journal

	MEAL I ATE	MY MOOD	HOW IT MADE ME FEEL	OTHER THINGS I NOTICED
BREAKFAST				
LUNCH				
SNACK				
DINNER				

Food & Feel Journal

	MEAL I ATE	MY MOOD	HOW IT MADE ME FEEL	OTHER THINGS I NOTICED
BREAKFAST				
LUNCH				
SNACK				
DINNER				

Food & Feel Journal

	MEAL I ATE	MY MOOD	HOW IT MADE ME FEEL	OTHER THINGS I NOTICED
BREAKFAST				
LUNCH				
SNACK				
DINNER				

Food & Feel Journal

	MEAL I ATE	MY MOOD	HOW IT MADE ME FEEL	OTHER THINGS I NOTICED
BREAKFAST				
LUNCH				
SNACK				
DINNER				

Food & Feel Journal

	MEAL I ATE	MY MOOD	HOW IT MADE ME FEEL	OTHER THINGS I NOTICED
BREAKFAST				
LUNCH				
SNACK				
DINNER				

Food & Feel Journal

	MEAL I ATE	MY MOOD	HOW IT MADE ME FEEL	OTHER THINGS I NOTICED
BREAKFAST				
LUNCH				
SNACK				
DINNER				

Food & Feel Journal

	MEAL I ATE	MY MOOD	HOW IT MADE ME FEEL	OTHER THINGS I NOTICED
BREAKFAST				
LUNCH				
SNACK				
DINNER				

Food & Feel Journal

	MEAL I ATE	MY MOOD	HOW IT MADE ME FEEL	OTHER THINGS I NOTICED
BREAKFAST				
LUNCH				
SNACK				
DINNER				

Food & Feel Journal

	MEAL I ATE	MY MOOD	HOW IT MADE ME FEEL	OTHER THINGS I NOTICED
BREAKFAST				
LUNCH				
SNACK				
DINNER				

Food & Feel Journal

	MEAL I ATE	MY MOOD	HOW IT MADE ME FEEL	OTHER THINGS I NOTICED
BREAKFAST				
LUNCH				
SNACK				
DINNER				

Food & Feel Journal

	MEAL I ATE	MY MOOD	HOW IT MADE ME FEEL	OTHER THINGS I NOTICED
BREAKFAST				
LUNCH				
SNACK				
DINNER				

Food & Feel Journal

	MEAL I ATE	MY MOOD	HOW IT MADE ME FEEL	OTHER THINGS I NOTICED
BREAKFAST				
LUNCH				
SNACK				
DINNER				

Notes

Notes

Notes

References

1) An International Journal of Medicine, Volume 95, Issue 9, September 2002, Pages 559-569, https://doi.org/10.1093/qjmed/95.9.559

2) Department of Gastroenterology and Hepatology, Yokohama City University Graduate School of Medicine, Yokohama, Japan, 2017, Efficacy of glutathione for the treatment of nonalcoholic fatty liver disease: an open-label, single-arm, multicenter, pilot study, volume 17, page 1.

3) Dr. Siri Carpenter, American Psychological Association, September 2012, Vol 43, No. 8, https://www.apa.org/monitor/2012/09/gut-feeling

4) Mayo Clinic, Hypothyroidism (Underactive Thyroid), Nov. 19, 2020, https://www.mayoclinic.org/diseases-conditions/hypothyroidism/symptoms-causes/syc-20350284

5) Mayo Clinic, Hashimoto's Disease, Feb. 11, 2020, https://www.mayoclinic.org/diseases-conditions/hashimotos-disease/symptoms-causes/syc-20351855

6) Mayo Clinic, https://www.mayoclinic.org/diseases-conditions/graves-disease/symptoms-causes/syc-20356240

7) National Institute of Health Office of Dietary Supplements, Vitamin D Fact Sheet for Health Professionals, March 2021, https://ods.od.nih.gov/factsheets/VitaminD-HealthProfessional/

8) Mary-Line Jugan, et al, November 2009, Endocrine Disruptors and Thyroid Hormones, https://www.sciencedirect.com/science/article/abs/pii/S0006295209009708

9) Valeria Calsolario, et al, Int. J. Mol. Sci. 2017, 18(12), 2583; https://doi.org/10.3390/ijms18122583, https://www.mdpi.com/1422-0067/18/12/2583/htm

10) Adrian Man, etal, Antimicrobial Activity of Six Essential Oils Against a Group of Human Pathogens: A Comparative Study, 2019 Jan 28. doi: 10.3390/pathogens8010015, https://www.ncbi.nlm.nih.gov/pmc/articles/PMC6471180/

11) Center for Disease Control, SKIN EXPOSURES & EFFECTS, https://www.cdc.gov/niosh/topics/skin/default.html

References

12) Center for Disease Control, Per-and Polyflourinated Substances (PFAS) Fact Sheet, https://www.cdc.gov/biomonitoring/PFAS_FactSheet.html

13) Hormone Health Network, November 2018, https://www.hormone.org/your-health-and-hormones/glands-and-hormones-a-to-z/hormones/cortisol

14) Journal of Thyroid Research: Ana Paula and Tania Weber Fulanetto, Role of Estrogen in Thyroid Function and Growth Regulation, 2011, https://www.ncbi.nlm.nih.gov/pmc/articles/PMC3113168/

15) J J Michnovicz and H L Bradlow, (1991), Altered estrogen metabolism and excretion in humans following consumption of indole-3-carbinol, Nutrition and Cancer, 16(1):59-66. doi: 10.1080/01635589109514141, https://pubmed.ncbi.nlm.nih.gov/1656396/

16) Melanie H. Jacobson et al, (2018 Mar 8), Paediatric and Perinatal Epidemiology, Thyroid hormones and menstrual cycle function in a longitudinal cohort of premenopausal women, https://www.ncbi.nlm.nih.gov/pmc/articles/PMC5980701/

17) Nangia Sangita Ajmanie, et al (2016), Role of Thyroid Dysfunction in Patients with Menstrual Disorders in Tertiary Care Center of Walled City of Delhi, J Obstet Gynaecol India, 66(2): 115-119, https://www.ncbi.nlm.nih.gov/pmc/articles/PMC4818825/

18) M Palmery et al, (2013 Jul), Oral contraceptives and changes in nutritional requirements, Eur Rev Med Pharmacol Sci., 17(13):1804-13. https://pubmed.ncbi.nlm.nih.gov/23852908/

19) Magdalena Tmoszuk et al, (August 2018), Evening Primrose (Oenothera biennis) Biological Activity Dependent on Chemical Composition, Antioxidants, 7(8): 108, https://www.ncbi.nlm.nih.gov/pmc/articles/PMC6116039/

20) Kanti Bhooshan Pandey et al, (2009), Plant polyphenols as dietary antioxidants in human health and disease, Oxidative Medicine and Cellular Longevity, 2(5): 270-278, https://www.ncbi.nlm.nih.gov/pmc/articles/PMC2835915/

21) Rosário Monteiro et l, (2014), Estrogen Signaling in Metabolic Inflammation, Mediators of Inflammation, doi: 10.1155/2014/615917, https://www.ncbi.nlm.nih.gov/pmc/articles/PMC4226184/

References

22) Luoping Zhang et al, (2009), Exposure to Glyphosate-Based Herbicides and Risk for Non-Hodgkin Lymphoma: A Meta-Analysis and Supporting Evidence, Mutation Research, 781: 186-206, https://www.ncbi.nlm.nih.gov/pmc/articles/PMC6706269/

23) A Wayne Meikle, (2004), The interrelationships between thyroid dysfunction and hypogonadism in men and boys, Thyroid, 14 Suppl 1:S17-25, https://pubmed.ncbi.nlm.nih.gov/15142373/

24) Peter H Bisschop et al, (2006), The effects of sex-steroid administration on the pituitary-thyroid axis in transsexuals, Eur J Endocrinol, 155(1):11-6, https://pubmed.ncbi.nlm.nih.gov/16793944/

25) Liselle Douyon et al, (2002), Effect of obesity and starvation on thyroid hormone, growth hormone, and cortisol secretion, Endocrinol Metab Clin North Am, 31(1):173-89, https://pubmed.ncbi.nlm.nih.gov/12055988/

26) Anthony C Hackney et al, (2009), Thyroid hormones and the interrelationship of cortisol and prolactin: influence of prolonged, exhaustive exercise, Endokrynol Pol, 60(4):252-7, https://pubmed.ncbi.nlm.nih.gov/19753538/

27) National Institute of General Medical Sciences, Circadian Rhythms, https://www.nigms.nih.gov/education/fact-sheets/Pages/circadian-rhythms.aspx

28) M. Nathaniel Mead, (2008), Benefits of Sunlight: A Bright Spot for Human Health, Environmental Health Perspectives, 116(4): A160-A167, https://www.ncbi.nlm.nih.gov/pmc/articles/PMC2290997/

29) Samih A Odhaib et al, (2019), How Biotin Induces Misleading Results in Thyroid Bioassays: Case Series, Cureus, 11(5): e4727, https://www.ncbi.nlm.nih.gov/pmc/articles/PMC6663274/

30) Zuzanna Sabina Goluch-Koniuszy, (2016), Nutrition of women with hair loss problem during the period of menopause, Menopause Review, 15(1): 56-61, https://www.ncbi.nlm.nih.gov/pmc/articles/PMC4828511/

31) National Institutes of Health, Selenium Fact Sheet, https://ods.od.nih.gov/factsheets/Selenium-HealthProfessional/

References

32) Roland Gärtner et all, April 2002, Journal of Clinical Endocrinology and Metabolism, Selenium supplementation in patients with autoimmune thyroiditis decreases thyroid peroxidase antibodies concentrations, https://pubmed.ncbi.nlm.nih.gov/11932302/

33) Surya Pierce, MD, October 2011, University of Wisconsin School of Medicine and Public Health, Integrative Treatment of Hypothyroidism, pg 4

34) Juliana Soares Severo and Jennifer Morais, (April 2019), The Role of Zinc in Thyroid Hormones Metabolism, International Journal for Vitamin and Nutrition Research, 89(1-2):1-9, https://www.researchgate.net/publication/332425890_The_Role_of_Zinc_in_Thyroid_Hormones_Metabolism

35) Jane Higdon, Ph.D. et al, Linus Pauling Institute, Iron, 2001, https://lpi.oregonstate.edu/mic/minerals/iron

36) Amy Myers MD, Omega 3s-and Your Thyroid, 2009, https://www.amymyersmd.com/article/omega-3-thyroid/

37) Abdul Jabbar et al, (2008), Vitamin B12 deficiency common in primary hypothyroidism, J Pak Med Assoc., 58(5):258-61, https://pubmed.ncbi.nlm.nih.gov/18655403/

38) S W Spaulding et al, (1976), Effect of caloric restriction and dietary composition of serum T3 and reverse T3 in man, J Clin Endocrinol Metabolism, https://pubmed.ncbi.nlm.nih.gov/1249190/

39) H. Tapiero et al, (Nov 2003), Trace elements in human physiology and pathology. Copper, Biomed Pharmacother. 57(9): 386-398, https://www.ncbi.nlm.nih.gov/pmc/articles/PMC6361146/

40) Manisha Arora et al, (July 5, 2018), Study of Trace Elements in Patients of Hypothyroidism with Special Reference to Zinc and Copper, https://biomedres.us/pdfs/BJSTR.MS.ID.001336.pdf

41) Dr. Amal Mohammed Husein Mackawy et al, (Nov 2013), Vitamin D Deficiency and Its Association with Thyroid Disease, International Journal of Health Sciences, 7(3): 267-275, https://www.ncbi.nlm.nih.gov/pmc/articles/PMC3921055/

References

42) State Water Control Board, September 2020, California Water Boards, https://www.waterboards.ca.gov/drinking_water/certlic/drinkingwater/Fluoridation.html

43) American Thyroid Association, Patient Thyroid Information: Is fluoridated drinking water associated with a higher prevalence of hypothyroidism?, https://www.thyroid.org/patient-thyroid-information/ct-for-patients/volume-8-issue-6/vol-8-issue-6-p-3/

44) Jagminder K. Bajaj et al, (Jan 2016), Various Possible Toxicants Involved in Thyroid Dysfunction: A Review, Journal of Clinical and Diagnostic Research, 10(1): FE01-FE03, https://www.ncbi.nlm.nih.gov/pmc/articles/PMC4740614/

45) Peter Felker et al, Concentrations of thiocyanate and goitrin in human plasma, their precursor concentrations in brassica vegetables, and associated potential risk for hypothyroidism, Nutrition Reviews, 74(4):248-58, https://pubmed.ncbi.nlm.nih.gov/26946249/

46) Brad Heins- organic dairy scientist, 2021, Grass-fed cows produce healthier milk, https://extension.umn.edu/pasture-based-dairy/grass-fed-cows-produce-healthier-milk

47) Mark Messina and Geoffrey Redmond, 2006 Mar, Effects of soy protein and soybean isoflavones on thyroid function in healthy adults and hypothyroid patients: a review of the relevant literature, Thyroid 16(3):249-58, doi: 10.1089/thy.2006.16.249. https://pubmed.ncbi.nlm.nih.gov/16571087/

48) Harvard School of Health; Lectins, https://www.hsph.harvard.edu/nutritionsource/anti-nutrients/lectins/

49) Dominika Skolmowska and Dominika Głąbska, (May 2019), Analysis of Heme and Non-Heme Iron Intake and Iron Dietary Sources in Adolescent Menstruating Females in a National Polish Sample, Nutrients, 11(5): 1049, https://www.ncbi.nlm.nih.gov/pmc/articles/PMC6567869/

50) Ashok Kumar Sharma et al, (Mar 2018), Efficacy and Safety of Ashwagandha Root Extract in Subclinical Hypothyroid Patients: A Double-Blind, Randomized Placebo-Controlled Trial, J Altern Complement Med, 24(3):243-248, https://www.ncbi.nlm.nih.gov/pubmed/28829155

51) National Institute Of Health. Magnesium Fact Sheet for Health Professionals. https://ods.od.nih.gov/factsheets/Magnesium-HealthProfessional/

References

52) Ganesh Chandra Jagetia and Bharat B Aggarwal, (Jan 2007), "Spicing up" of the immune system by curcumin, J Clin Immunol, 27(1):19-35, https://www.ncbi.nlm.nih.gov/pubmed/17211725

53) Yeon-Ran Kim, September 2005, Immunomodulatory Activity of the Water Extract from Mushroom inonotus obliquus, Mycobiology. 33(3): 158-162.

54) Zhu X, Lin Z. Modulation of cytokines production, granzyme B and perforin in murine CIK cells by Ganoderma lucidum polysaccharides. Carbohydr Polym. 2006;63:188-97.

55) Christine A. Houghton et al, (2016), Sulforaphane and Other Nutrigenomic Nrf2 Activators: Can the Clinician's Expectation Be Matched by the Reality?, Oxidative Medicine and Cellular Longevity, 17857186, https://www.ncbi.nlm.nih.gov/pmc/articles/PMC4736808/

Made in the USA
Las Vegas, NV
26 April 2024

89162245R00142